Psychiatric Hospitalization of School-Age Children

Psychiatric Hospitalization of School-Age Children

By

Richard Dalton, M.D.
Associate Professor of Psychiatry and Pediatrics

Marc A. Forman, M.D.
Professor of Psychiatry and Pediatrics

Tulane University School of Medicine
New Orleans, Louisiana

American Psychiatric Press, Inc.

Washington, DC
London, England

Note: The authors have worked to ensure that all information in this book concerning drug dosages, schedules, and routes of administration is accurate as of the time of publication and consistent with standards set by the U.S. Food and Drug Administration and the general medical community. As medical research and practice advance, however, therapeutic standards may change. For this reason and because human and mechanical errors sometimes occur, we recommend that readers follow the advice of a physician who is directly involved in their care or the care of a member of their family.

Manufactured in the United States of America on acid-free paper.
94 93 92 4 3 2 1
First Edition

American Psychiatric Press, Inc.
1400 K Street, N.W., Washington, DC 20005

Library of Congress Cataloging-in-Publication Data
Dalton, Richard. 1949–
Psychiatric hospitalization of school-age children / by Richard Dalton. Marc A. Forman. —1st ed.
p. cm.
Includes bibliographical references and index.
ISBN 0-88048-424-1
1. Child psychotherapy—Residential treatment. 2. Mentally ill children—Hospital care. 3. Psychiatric hospital care. I. Forman. Marc A., 1935– . II. Title.
[DNLM: 1. Child, Hospitalized. 2. Hospitals, Psychiatric. 3. Hospitalization. 4. Mental Disorders—in infancy & childhood. 5. Mental Disorders—therapy. 6. Psychotherapy—in infancy & childhood. 7. Psychotherapy—methods. WS 350.2 D152p]
RJ504.5.D33 1992
362.2'1'0834—dc20
DNLM/DLC 91-47119
for Library of Congress CIP

British Library Cataloguing in Publication Data
A CIP record is available from the British Library.

Contents

Acknowledgments

We would like to thank the staff of the Children's Neuropsychiatric Inpatient Unit at Tulane University Hospital for their care of the children on the unit; Jorge H. Daruna, Ph.D., Dorothy Bolding, Dr.P.H., and Jane Woods, R.N., for their clinical teamwork; Joseph B. Green, M.D., and Martin Irwin, M.D., who planned and developed the Tulane unit; and Daniel K. Winstead, M.D., and hospital administration for their ongoing support of the program. The Kirschman Foundation and the New Orleans Institute of Mental Hygiene have generously provided funds for our overall child psychiatry program, and to them we extend our deepest appreciation. We also wish to acknowledge the contribution of the staff of the Children's Unit at New Orleans Adolescent Hospital, the assistance of the Office of Community Services, and other agencies with whom we have collaborated in Louisiana and Mississippi. Finally, we owe a special debt to Margot Young, who processed our words into a finished manuscript with grace and patience.

Foreword

In their incisive book, *Psychiatric Hospitalization of School-Age Children,* Richard Dalton and Marc Forman have brought order out of chaos. Each of the authors has brought to this volume separate experiences with troubled children, coming from differing vantage points to join forces in their dedication to filling children's psychiatric needs.

Richard Dalton has had a rich exposure to the stresses created by pediatric illness. His deep involvement in a children's burn unit at the University of North Carolina, and especially his responsibility for the psychologic program of a boy placed in a bubble at Duke University Hospital because of a congenital immune deficiency disease, made him much more than a routine child psychiatrist.

Marc Forman brings a unique background to the philosophy underlying this book. Schooled in the gallant but overwhelmed community mental health programs at St. Christopher's Hospital for Children and at Temple University, he learned how easily children are forgotten in the forging of brave plans. From then on, Dr. Forman dedicated himself to the psychiatric needs of children, with ever-growing responsibilities for both clinical care and administrative expertise.

Brought together at the Division of Child Psychiatry at Tulane University Medical Center, Drs. Dalton and Forman have distilled the essence of their varied careers. Using the venerated medical tradition of healing the few, relieving the pain of those who cannot be healed, and bringing comfort and understanding to the many, they have applied this maxim to troubled children and their families.

Infrequently there may come a time during the effort to intervene successfully into a child's circle of despair or alienation, when an out-of-hospital psychiatric approach cannot be productive. This inability to intervene successfully may be due to the nature of the psychiatric disorder itself or to extraordinarily inimical environmental factors. Or it may have its roots in a poor fit between the child's individual characteristics and the demands and expectations of the environment. In these cases, an inpatient locus for diagnosis and determination of effective intervention, especially for the youngster in middle childhood (i.e., the years between preschool and adolescence), is crucial. However, when inpatient care is required, the complex nature of the needs to be met simultaneously for each child on an inpatient unit, the requirement that there be an organized environment and schooling for the disorganized child, the necessity for containing aggression simultaneously with the essential task of comprehending the aggressive impulse—these and other factors make the nature of a hospital psychiatric unit for children in middle childhood a delicate structure.

While overall guides and rules are available, anyone who has had the experience of organizing any supposedly well-understood structure must be prepared to find unexpected pitfalls. This volume, *Psychiatric Hospitalization of School-Age Children,* especially fills this need. The authors, from the vantage point of a functioning hospital psychiatric service for children of the middle childhood years (ages 6 through 12), present and discuss a philosophy of treatment that is typically neither examined nor stated in other publications. It is based on an interactional (or transactional) model. This model underlies their concept of the indications for admission, for treatment plans, and for the organization of the milieu, as well as for the length of stay and discharge planning. The authors examine the ideas and opinions to be found in the extensive literature and balance them against the daily realities.

Although not a blueprint or a "how to" volume, this book is organized in such a way that it tracks the patient, the family, and the physician or mental health professional throughout the entire process from prehospitalization to posthospitalization. Although the discussion can be used to help with difficult decisions, the authors are well aware that circumstances and purposes differ and that, consequently, the shapes of inpatient units must differ accordingly.

The authors review treatment from mulitple perspectives in a nondiagnostic and nonideological fashion and consider most lucidly the place of hospitalization within the entire spectrum.

It is refreshing to find theoretical issues tied to practical considerations. There are many intrusive factors that prevent the carrying out of ideal plans. These factors, detailed in most of the book's chapters as "confounding issues," constitute a most useful series of red flags of warning. The authors are particularly concerned with interferences with continuity of effective treatment, including the confounding issues that prevent prehospitalization forging of alliances with parents or surrogate caregivers, the failure to locate appropriate but less restrictive circumstances to serve as steps toward competent return to the community, and precipitate admissions and discharges. And yet, while noting the confounding issues and itemizing the administrative pluses and minuses, the authors continue to provide an ideal against which can be judged each effort to help a foundering child and family through a period of hospital observation and therapeutic beginnings.

Of considerable help in converting a lofty ideal into a practical reality is the balanced discussion of contemporary economic factors that, in today's world, affect hospitalization.

This book is not an itemized pipe dream. It was written by physicians who know and respect children and also know and respect practicality. To flesh out this combination, we are given a number of vivid and pertinent case examples that bring to life real children being treated in a real hospital and coming from and returning to a real world.

Stella Chess, M.D.
Professor of Child Psychiatry
New York University Medical Center
New York, New York

Overview

It is the purpose of this book to provide an understanding of current clinical practice in inpatient psychiatric units for children in middle childhood (ages 6 to 12), as well as to present our opinion about what contemporary optimal care should be. To accomplish this goal we present our philosophy of treatment and its ramifications for the inpatient therapy process, a review of efficacy studies, and an in-depth discussion of the indications for admission. We then examine aspects of the hospitalization process itself, including diagnostic assessment, treatment planning, the phases of hospitalization, discharge planning, and aftercare. We describe the role of individual psychotherapy, the uses of behavioral techniques in discrete therapies as well as within the general milieu, group therapy and group dynamics, pharmacotherapy and its integration into the total treatment process, the various approaches to family therapy and parent training, and the treatment of special clinical problems and symptoms often seen in patients admitted to child inpatient units. We review the function of the milieu, the school program, and administrative and staff organization.

Within the microcosm of the hospital setting, inpatient care reflects all subject areas of contemporary child psychiatry: diagnosis; individual, family, behavioral, group and pharmacotherapies; use of allied health professionals and paraprofessionals; liaison to schools and pediatrics; and training, research, and administration. However in this volume, we limit our discussion to how these concerns relate specifically to hospitalization.

Furthermore, we outline those obstacles that confound delivery of optimal care within various inpatient settings (university hospitals, for-profit hospitals, state facilities, children's hospitals, etc.). While the complexities of inpatient psychiatric care for school-age children do not allow for a "how to" book, we hope that this volume provides a useful guide to those mental health professionals who are involved in the planning, organization, or administration of inpatient units, as well as those who participate in direct clinical care.

Richard Dalton, M.D.
Marc A. Forman, M.D.

Chapter 1

Historical Perspectives

To understand contemporary inpatient child psychiatry we must first examine the historical antecedents that have influenced the development of current theory and practice (Table 1–1). Our chronological perspective begins in the 18th century, by which time the slow change from feudalism to life in the cities had created a population of both delinquent and parentless children. Orphanages were established to provide for their care. Although initially custodial in nature, the care provided in orphanages was subsequently affected by changes in social philosophy during the mid-18th century. The nascent social consciousness developing at that time, which influenced care offered in penal, educational, and medical institutions, helped change the emphasis within orphanages from custodial care to rehabilitation and education (Aichorn 1939).

The European humanistic movement, derived from the philosophy of John Locke (who emphasized the rational aspects of human nature, the importance of the environment, and the need for knowledge to be based in science rather than dogma), influenced the fields of education and psychiatry and contributed very positively to these social changes. Vilain's introduction of orderly ways of treating inmates, Howard's development of family-like cottages within orphanages, Pinel's unshackling of severely disturbed patients, and Itard's description of his treatment of a feral boy (Stone 1979) were examples of this movement. Its growing effect was seen in the flexible educational environments advocated by Rousseau and Pestalozzi and in Froebel's establishment of the first kindergarten. People began to view children as having their own development and personalities as opposed to the previously held notion of children as miniature adults.

The 19th century witnessed additional advances in the understanding of human development leading to the incorporation of two novel ideas into the educational movement: first, that children's spontaneous activities are important in the educational process; and, second, that children pass through definite developmental stages that influence later learning. The

Table 1–1. The historical antecedents that have influenced the development of current theory and practice in inpatient child psychiatry

1700s	Orphanages established to provide care for the population of both delinquent and parentless children that had resulted, in part, from the slow change from feudalism toward urbanization.
Mid-1700s	Changes in social philosophy helped to change the emphasis within orphanages from custodial care to rehabilitation and education. People began to view children as having their own development and personalities as opposed to the previously held notion of children as miniature adults.
1800s	Further understanding of human (and specifically child) development led to further acceptance of childhood as an entity per se. Children were found to pass through definite developmental stages that influence later learning. Children's spontaneous activities were determined to be important in the educational process.
Late 1800s	Institutions created in the United States for children with special needs.
	Precursors of *child guidance movement* underway as characterized by progressive developments in social reform, juvenile delinquency, and education.
Early 1900s	Establishment of juvenile courts associated with a new approach that considered the child's motivation for a delinquent act and assessed the best disposition for the child rather than determining guilt. Courts given permission to remove children from deleterious home environments and to place them in foster homes, in residential facilities, and, later, in hospitals.
	Advent of intellectual and psychological testing associated with shift in focus on problem children from identification and containment to treatment and remediation.
	Dynamic psychiatry attempted to distinguish individual types of mental illness by using history, symptoms, and behaviors as a means of differentiation. The importance of biographical data and, subsequently, developmental information in searching for the causes of psychological illness emphasized by Freud and Meyer.
	The concept of preventive medicine within the arena of mental health advanced by the *mental hygiene movement,* fortified by changes within the public health movement (e.g., advances in bacteriology). Emphasis on understanding childhood symptoms as opposed to treating them punitively.

Table 1–1. The historical antecedents that have influenced the development of current theory and practice in inpatient child psychiatry (continued)

	First child psychiatry inpatient units established (e.g., at Bellevue and Kingsport hospitals in New York). Although initially managerial, the treatment objectives of these units subsequently drew from the child guidance and residential facility movements and quickly influenced inpatient services.
Mid-1900s	Principles of psychoanalysis and ego psychology applied to the therapy of nonorganically impaired patients in various diagnostic categories.
	Lengths of stay extended, emphasis placed on individual psychotherapy, and administrative format changed to place the individual therapist in charge of case.
	Introduction of systems theory during the 1960s, leading to the growth of family therapy and milieu therapy.
	Advances in biological psychiatry and psychopharmacology (e.g., neuroleptics, antidepressants, antianxiety agents, anticonvulsants) dramatically affected inpatient care.
	Behavioral principles incorporated into the milieu, parent training, and individual therapy.
Late 1900s	Understanding the neural correlates of behavior, which has changed the way patients' symptoms are viewed.
	National economic and social forces have led to alterations in patient population, treatment practices, and treatment philosophy. Constraints set by third-party payers have shortened lengths of stay.
	The growth of inpatient units within for-profit hospitals during the 1970s and 1980s has influenced admission criteria, patient-staff ratios, and transitions to and from the hospital.
	Social issues (e.g., the disorganization of family life) shift current patient type toward more aggressive children and children with conduct disorder, who often have been subjected to abuse and neglect and are not living with both biological parents. Lengths of stay have decreased, interfering with traditional inpatient alliance building and the establishment of trust. Accordingly, physical limit setting occupies a greater portion of staff energy and time.
	Many inpatient therapists now appear satisfied with symptom reduction as opposed to laying the groundwork for continued developmental growth and substantive psychological change.

publication of numerous books describing early development furthered the acceptance of childhood as an entity per se. Edouard Seguin applied these new educational principles while working with mentally retarded and psychologically disturbed children in Paris and, later, in the United States. By 1876, there were eight institutions in seven states within this country caring for 1,300 children with special needs (Lowrey 1945).

The entrance of psychologists onto the scene early in the 20th century furthered the cause of the humanists. With the advent of intellectual and psychological testing, educational and medical professionals (and, later, the general public) began to focus not only on identifying and containing problem children, but also on treatment and remediation. Binet's study of psychometry in Paris along with Goddard's introduction of these tests into the United States represented critical steps in this process (Stone 1979).

By the late 19th and early 20th centuries, continued progressive developments in social reform, juvenile delinquency, and education led, in part, to the creation of the *child guidance movement,* which, more than any other single event, led to the formation of child psychiatry as a unique professional discipline (Hetznecker and Forman 1971). The child guidance philosophy determined the type of care offered within residential facilities, which had evolved by the early 20th century from their beginnings as orphanages.

At the same time, dynamic psychiatry was attempting to distinguish individual types of mental illness by using history, symptoms, and behaviors as a means of differentiation. Freud and Meyer emphasized the importance of biographical data and, subsequently, developmental information in searching for the causes of psychological illness.

The *mental hygiene movement,* fortified by changes within the public health movement (e.g., advances in bacteriology), advanced the concept of preventive medicine within the arena of mental health. This concept was applied to psychiatric maladies by the second decade of this century. This preventive approach emphasized understanding childhood symptoms as opposed to treating them punitively.

The establishment of the first juvenile court in 1899 heralded a new approach in which judges reviewed the child's motivation for a delinquent act and were more concerned about making the best disposition for the child rather than determining guilt (Hetznecker and Forman 1971). Courts were given permission to remove children from deleterious home environments and to place them in foster homes, in residential facilities, and, later, in hospitals.

In short, the interest in human welfare that burgeoned during the 18th century positively affected the understanding and treatment of children during the 19th and 20th centuries. Care in orphanages and residential facilities changed accordingly. Psychological theories of motivation were proffered and treatment strategies were developed and applied.

The first child psychiatry inpatient units were established at Bellevue and Kingsport hospitals in New York, at the Franklin School in Pennsylvania during the late 1920s, and at Bradley Hospital in Rhode Island during the early 1930s to treat and manage postencephalitic children with severe behavioral disorders (Barker 1974). Although the treatment objectives of these units were initially managerial, the therapeutic philosophy subsequently adopted from the child guidance and residential facility movements quickly influenced inpatient services (Hersov and Bentovim 1985).

The scope of treatment offered on inpatient units broadened during the 1940s and 1950s as the principles of psychoanalysis and ego psychology were applied to the therapy of nonorganically impaired patients in various diagnostic categories. This approach went hand in hand with the accepted tenets of inpatient care during that era: extended lengths of stay, emphasis on individual psychotherapy, and an administrative format in which the individual therapist was invariably in charge of the case. The introduction of systems theory during the 1960s led to the growth of family therapy and milieu therapy, and challenged the traditional views about what was important regarding inpatient care. Although some hospitals and therapists had long recognized the utility of these new approaches, they were accepted into general practice only after a fair amount of acrimonious debate.

Subsequent advances in biological psychiatry and psychopharmacology dramatically affected inpatient care. Neuroleptic agents significantly altered the treatment of psychotic children during the 1960s and 1970s, and antidepressant, antianxiety, and anticonvulsant drugs have extended our ability to treat other disorders. Just as important, however, has been our understanding of the neural correlates of behavior, which has changed the way in which we now view patient symptoms. Furthermore the incorporation of behavioral principles, initially resisted by some practitioners, has guided strategies used in the milieu, parent training, and individual therapy. Social learning theory and specific behavioral therapy techniques are now widely employed by inpatient therapists in their work with children and parents.

More recent national economic and social forces have led to alterations in patient population, treatment practices, and treatment philosophy. Contemporary constraints set by third-party payers have significantly affected the operation of inpatient units during the past 15 years, exerting considerable pressure toward shortened lengths of stay. As a counterpoint, the growth of inpatient units within for-profit hospitals during the 1970s and 1980s has influenced admission criteria, patient-staff ratios, and transitions to and from the hospital.

Social issues, especially those that reflect the unfortunate disorganization of family life, have also had their impact. A review by Jemerin and

Philips (1988) of changes on their inpatient unit between 1975 and 1985 is similar to our own experience and underscores recent national trends. They note a marked shift in current patient type toward more aggressive children and children with conduct disorder, who often have been subjected to abuse and neglect and are not living with both biological parents. Many of their patients are now within state custody, complicating both payment for services and posthospitalization disposition and placement. Lengths of stay have decreased, interfering with traditional inpatient alliance building and the establishment of trust. Patient management techniques within the milieu have been altered accordingly. Because of decreasing lengths of stay combined with the increase in physical aggression by patients, physical limit setting has occupied a greater portion of staff energy and time. Medications are used more liberally. Disorganized families are harder to engage in the treatment process, and, associated with the shortened lengths of stay, many do not receive the type of attention needed to mitigate a recurrence of symptoms following discharge. On some units the therapeutic emphasis has shifted dramatically from individual therapy and patient-oriented issues to control within the milieu, placing added stress on unit and nursing personnel. Jemerin and Philips suggest that hospitalization goals have changed. Many inpatient therapists now appear satisfied with symptom reduction as opposed to laying the groundwork for continued developmental growth and substantive psychological change (see Chapter 2).

References

Aichorn A: Wayward Youth. New York, Viking, 1939

Barker P: History, in The Residential Psychiatric Treatment of Children. Edited by Barker P. New York, Wiley, 1974, pp 1–26

Hersov L, Bentovim A: Inpatient and day-hospital units, in Child and Adolescent Psychiatry: Modern Approaches, 2nd Edition. Edited by Rutter M, Hersov L. Oxford, UK, Blackwell Scientific, 1985, pp 766–779

Hetznecker W, Forman MA: Community child psychiatry: evolution and direction. Am J Orthopsychiatry 41:350–370, 1971

Jemerin JM, Philips I: Changes in inpatient child psychiatry: consequences and recommendations. J Am Acad Child Adolesc Psychiatry 27:397–403, 1988

Lowrey L: Psychiatry for children. Am J Psychiatry 101:375–388, 1945

Stone LA: Residential treatment, in Basic Handbook of Child Psychiatry, Vol 3: Therapeutic Interventions. Edited by Harrison SI (JD Noshpitz, Editor-in-Chief). New York, Basic Books, 1979, pp 231–262

Chapter 2

Philosophy of Treatment

Philosophy of treatment refers to the theoretical view of what the therapeutic process can potentially offer the patient. There are three generally held notions about what can actually result from therapy (Table 2–1). Each has been used as a basis for designing therapeutic approaches to patient problems.

The first, *symptom reduction or relief,* underscores the principle that therapy should be seen as a means of helping the patient manage primary complaints and presenting behaviors. Once done, the therapy process has achieved its purpose and termination should result. The second philosophical approach, which involves the *notion of cure,* implies that the presenting complaints and symptoms represent the tip of the iceberg; thus, therapeutic techniques and strategies should be directed toward underlying dynamics designed to significantly change the individual's personality. The third view of therapy holds that the key element involves *improvement of the "fit" between the child and the interpersonal environment.* The underlying implication is that after the child and environment are more appropriately attuned, reasonable developmental growth will ensue.

The transactional risk model, most recently elaborated by Woolston (1989), best describes this third example of treatment philosophy. In this model the following are examined:

1. The individual child—the child's self, including temperament and proclivities toward genetic illnesses, impulsivity, and hyperactivity; the sense of self, including both devalued and idealized internalizations; and the sense of others
2. The child's internal mechanisms that are used to understand and react to the environment (e.g., perceptions, intelligence, integrating mechanisms, defense mechanisms, judgment, reality testing)
3. The environment itself, including the overall condition of the environment and particular stressful events and times

4. The intrapsychic representations and mechanisms of significant others in the environment

Most important, the model clarifies the relationship among these components and seeks to determine how they fit together. Researchers are currently studying the relationship between child and environment by examining these variables (Chess and Thomas 1984; Jones 1986).

This work is important because it helps to crystallize specific areas requiring attention during the therapeutic process. Whereas the treatment philosophy calling for cure implies that therapeutic attention should be directed toward the child's self system and perception of self, the transactional model emphasizes the importance of evaluating the child within the environment so that therapeutic emphasis can be directed variously toward the child's self system or perceptual system, toward family members' self systems or perceptual systems, and to the interaction among the systems, as well as to the environment itself. The choice of emphasis depends on the most notable areas of weakness. The guiding principle is that a more favorable alignment between child and interpersonal environment is, in and of itself, therapeutic.

Accepted inpatient treatment philosophy has changed through the years. During the 1920s and 1930s, hospitalization was designed to relieve symptoms. From the 1940s to the 1970s, when the psychoanalytic model was so influential in guiding inpatient work, treatment philosophy involved the concept of cure. Since then, changes have occurred. Although not well

Table 2–1. Three generally held notions underlying treatment

Symptom reduction or relief	Underscores the principle that therapy should be seen as a means of helping the patient manage primary complaints and presenting behaviors. Once done, the therapy process has achieved its purpose and termination should result.
Cure	The presenting complaints and symptoms represent the tip of the iceberg; thus, therapeutic techniques and strategies should be directed toward underlying dynamics designed to significantly change the individual's personality.
Improvement of the "fit" between the child and the interpersonal environment (transactional risk model)	Underlying implication is that after the child and environment are more appropriately attuned, reasonable developmental growth will ensue.

formulated for quite some time, the currently accepted notion is that the child should be treated until factors have changed sufficiently so that discharge to a less restrictive setting (usually back home) is possible without the type of symptom recurrence that would require rehospitalization or seriously hamper long-term development. The transactional risk model is the theoretical force underlying this current view, and we have found it to be the most coherent, practical, effective model for our inpatient work.

What naturally follows from this treatment philosophy is a multifocused evaluation and treatment approach directed toward each intrapsychic, interpersonal, and environmental factor contributing to the patient's problems. To accomplish this, inpatient units must be prepared to provide the specific therapies—individual, family, behavioral, group, and biological—necessary to appropriately manage particular situations. Furthermore, this model necessitates certain considerations regarding the admission and evaluation processes, treatment planning, and the maintenance of a positive milieu, as well as the use of research and follow-up data.

Goals for Hospitalization

Goals for hospitalization are often erroneously equated with philosophy. Actually, the former, which define what the treatment team wants to accomplish as a result of its various therapies, flow naturally from philosophy. When the accepted philosophical approach was to strive for cure, goals specified necessary intrapsychic changes (reconstruction of personality variables leading to substantive ego changes). When the approach was to strive for symptom reduction, goals were behavioral (stabilization of the patient). With the transactional model in mind, we think that current inpatient treatment goals should include

1. The evaluation of the critical areas within the previously described fit—or, more appropriately, "mis-fit"—between child and interpersonal environment that are contributing to the problems
2. The direction of therapeutic energies to the particular aspect(s) of the mis-fit that must change to allow for patient stabilization and subsequent transfer to a less restrictive setting as soon as possible without unduly negative consequences for developmental growth
3. The provision of a safe, secure environment that encourages healthy interaction and change
4. The development of a treatment plan that reflects a thorough understanding of long-term needs and uses therapeutic techniques that can be adapted to a posthospitalization therapy program for satisfaction of those needs.

Length of Stay

The transactional risk model and the goals mentioned above do not predetermine the type of therapies used in any particular hospitalization, nor do they solely dictate length of stay. In those cases when very brief, specifically directed inpatient therapies can attune the child and interpersonal environment sufficiently so that posthospitalization treatment can successfully accomplish long-term goals, hospitalization and interventions should be focused and brief. However, in those cases when the necessary ingredients for attuning the fit do not readily come together so that continued improvement in a less restrictive setting is not possible, medium- or long-term inpatient care is appropriate and in-depth hospital treatment is required. In this model, what really differentiates long-term from short-term work are pragmatic issues (e.g., levels of patient and family pathology and strengths, less restrictive treatment settings available that can fulfill long-term patient goals) associated with each particular case and situation.

Investigators have attempted to elucidate the variables contributing to length of stay. Over 20 factors have been identified as possibly contributing to extensiveness of hospitalization for adults, including psychiatric condition, posthospitalization support (Mezzich and Coffman 1985), and specific treatment variables (Cyr and Haley 1983). Regarding child and adolescent lengths of stay, Forness and colleagues (1985) have concluded that diagnosis alone is not a predictor. Some authors have suggested that low intelligence and autistic symptoms are correlated (Oliver and Knight 1984), while others (Gordon et al. 1985) have found the Axis IV–to–Axis V ratio to be predictive (although their supporting data are not compelling). Christ et al. (1989) have related length of stay to the type of hospital (public versus private) and service offered (short-term versus long-term).

Our own experience is that the length of a patient's stay is dependent on a number of patient, family, and treatment variables (Ward et al. 1991). On our university unit, length of stay correlates with discharge placement problems (see Chapter 6) and a history of parental delinquent behavior. On our state hospital unit, where length of stay is much longer, even when socioeconomic and third-party payer issues are controlled for, extensiveness of hospitalization is correlated with severity of behavior problems, as well as a plethora of treatment and administrative issues (e.g., low staff-patient ratio, reduced number of therapy sessions per week, increased amount of paperwork).

Generally, we think that a period of at least 3 to 4 weeks is necessary for the treatment of children with serious anxiety disorders and favorably responding affective disorders. A period of at least 6 weeks is required for treating children with aggressive conduct disorders and (developing) characterological problems. A greater amount of time is often necessary for treating psychotic and organically impaired children. Although generally accepted (Brugger 1990), these guidelines should not be rigidly enforced. We think that those short-term units with rather brief, predetermined lengths of stay (Doherty et al. 1987) run the risk of inadequately treating seriously disturbed, aggressive, and psychotic patients.

Case Example

Dave, a 10-year-old, was admitted to our university unit after he sexually molested a 3-year-old boy in his foster home. The patient had been encopretic and enuretic on a daily basis for over a year and was frequently aggressive and violent at school. Dave had been taken into state custody at 8 years of age when it was discovered that his mother's boyfriend was repeatedly involving him in oral and anal sexual activities. Although the symptoms mentioned above were present at that time, they seriously worsened after he was sexually abused by a boy in his first foster home placement. He was then hospitalized in a state facility for symptom stabilization where his principle treatment consisted of group and pharmacological therapies. He was discharged after his aggression and sexual acting out were fairly well controlled; however, his encopresis and enuresis continued unabated.

Dave was placed in a residential facility following hospitalization with no follow-up therapy. His symptoms slowly returned until, several months later, he was transferred to a foster home (again without therapy) with the hope that a family setting would help him feel more secure. He was hospitalized after his sexual acting out with the foster parents' 3-year-old biological son was discovered. During our evaluation, it was determined that he suffered with a posttraumatic stress disorder, in addition to obvious behavioral and developing characterological problems. Dave's aggressive acting out, encopresis, and enuresis remitted within the first 3 weeks of admission. It was clear, however, that without skilled therapy, support, and environmental structure, his problematic behaviors would readily return until he became able to acknowledge what had actually happened to him in the past and to begin to deal with his subsequently developed feelings. Because of the unavailability of less restrictive facilities in the public sector capable of providing the therapies needed within a supportive environment, Dave's hospitalization was extended for 5 months until his self-related conflicts could be sufficiently treated so that continued developmental progress within the available, least restrictive level of care would be possible. At discharge he was moved into another foster home, after a planned transition, and continued in twice-per-week outpatient individual therapy with his hospital therapist.

This case exemplifies how medium- to long-term inpatient care is a product of patient, treatment, and environmental factors. Dave's self system was modified in a positive direction once we helped him therapeutically face his past sexual abuse. This work, occurring within an inpatient environment, enabled him to "fit" into a carefully chosen foster care environment, where therapy could continue. If there had been a therapeutic foster home, group home, or residential facility able to supportively manage his symptoms during the therapy process, the length of stay could have been significantly shorter. What could have been long-term, outpatient treatment goals (e.g., the development of trust, therapeutic discussion of past events, emotional abreaction) became hospitalization goals by default.

Confounding Issues

The transactional model and our subsequently developed goals for hospitalization do not tell the whole story, however. What is important is not that clinicians necessarily adhere to this particular treatment philosophy, but that they adopt and examine their own models regarding what ought to happen during hospitalization and that these models be based on what is in the patient's best interest. One cannot work without a philosophy of treatment. Clinicians must understand and comprehend the nature of the task. Without an (at least) implicitly conscious model, clinicians are less likely to operate within a consistently coherent plan. This is often the main problem with clinicians who are not adequately trained to do this work.

As discussed in the previous chapter, recent social and economic changes have contributed to the changing character of both individual patients (i.e., harder to manage) and inpatient length of stay (decreasing length of stay along with increasingly used managed care). This combination has led some units to abandon the transactional model in favor of the more readily (and easily) accomplishable goals associated with symptom reduction. We think that this leads to ineffective care, except when very specific self-related issues are responsible for the mis-fit between child and environment. In addition, economically generated issues, especially the underlying profit motives of providers, might, either directly or indirectly, negatively influence the delivery of care as well as the indications used for the admission and discharge of patients. (We examine the issues related to managed care in Chapter 15 and those related to the economic factors mentioned above in Chapter 4.)

References

Brugger T: Child psychiatric hospitalization today: issues and problems. Paper presented at the 37th annual meeting of the American Academy of Child and Adolescent Psychiatry, Chicago, IL, October 1990

Chess S, Thomas A: Origins and Evolution of Behavior Disorder From Infancy to Early Adult Life. New York, Brunner/Mazel, 1984

Christ AE, Tsemberis S, Andrews H: Childhood disorder DRG: consideration for a predictive model. J Am Acad Child Adolesc Psychiatry 28:47–52, 1989

Cyr JJ, Haley GA: Use of demographic and clinical characteristics in predicting length of psychiatric hospital stay: a final evaluation. J Consult Clin Psychol 51:637–640, 1983

Doherty MB, Manderson M, Carter-Ake L: Time-limited psychiatric hospitalization of children: a model and three-year outcome. Hosp Community Psychiatry 38:643–647, 1987

Forness SR, Sinclair E, Alexson J, et al: Toward diagnostic related groups in child psychiatry: a preliminary study. J Am Acad Child Adolesc Psychiatry 24:266–272, 1985

Gordon RE, Jardiolin P, Gordon KK: Predicting length of hospital stay of psychiatric patients. Am J Psychiatry 142:235–237, 1985

Jones E: Interpreting interpersonal behavior. Science 234:41–46, 1986

Mezzich JE, Coffman GA: Factors influencing length of hospital stay. Hosp Community Psychiatry 36:1262–1264, 1270, 1985

Oliver J, Knight D: An evaluation of an inpatient psychiatric unit for children. Child: Care, Health, and Development 10:141–155, 1984

Ward K, Dalton R, Daruna J: Length of stay on latency-aged units. Paper presented at the annual meeting of the American Psychiatric Association, New Orleans, LA, May 1991

Woolston JL: Transactional risk model for short and intermediate term psychiatric inpatient treatment of children. J Am Acad Child Adolesc Psychiatry 28:38–41, 1989

Chapter 3

Efficacy Studies: A Review

Recent pressures within the field of mental health have raised questions about the appropriateness of psychiatric hospitalization for children, especially since its use for children is decreasing in other countries (Östman 1988). Increased scrutiny has underscored the need for efficacy studies to determine the utility of this level of care (Blotcky et al. 1984; Dalton et al. 1989). In this chapter we review and discuss currently available efficacy studies examining outcome of patients psychiatrically hospitalized on long-term and short-term school-age units. We also examine the type of research possible on inpatient units and discuss related issues.

To date, there are 46 studies examining the outcome of both traditional (primarily long-term) and short-term hospitalization. Blotcky and colleagues (1984) have previously reported on 24 of these efficacy studies, commenting on trends noted as well as specific research designs and statistical techniques used. We briefly examine their results, as well as selected data from the other 21 studies.

Forty studies have examined outcome following hospitalization on traditional units (see Table 3–1), while six studies have examined outcome following hospitalization on short-term units (Table 3–2). The potential conclusions that can be drawn from these studies are limited by the techniques used for gathering, analyzing, and reporting the data. Thirty-five of the 46 studies were retrospective. Seventeen used previously validated rating scales of patient behavior, and only 11 of them applied the ratings to behavior before and after hospitalization. Just 4 of the 46 studies were well controlled, and only 12 used contemporary statistical approaches to analyze data. Furthermore, 15 of the studies included adolescents.

Several problems are created by the methodological approaches used in these studies. The main shortcoming with retrospective studies is that charts rarely provide consistently usable, detailed information about patient and family behavior and treatment team approach. Without validated rating scales of behavior, before and after hospital treatment, it is difficult both to objectively measure patient change and to compare patients among studies. Furthermore, without adequately controlling for normative developmental progress, it is difficult to know whether the behavior measured at follow-up is a product of treatment or of expected developmental growth and change. In addition, the inclusion of adolescents raises serious questions about the usefulness of the results for latency-age children. Finally, without contemporary statistical approaches, it is very difficult to compare individual variables with each other as well as with variable clusters, which seriously limits possible conclusions.

In spite of the aforementioned shortcomings, these studies do produce useful information about the relationship between patient and family variables and outcome (Blotcky et al. 1984). Nine studies have attempted to correlate intelligence with outcome. Seven of them have concluded that

Table 3–1. Efficacy studies (through 1990) that have examined outcome of traditional (primarily long-term) hospitalization

1930s through the 1960s
(in chronological order)

- Rosenthal and Pinsky 1936
- Zick 1943
- Morris et al. 1956
- Kane and Chambers 1961
- Lawder and Nordan 1963
- Johnson and Rubin 1964
- Allerhand et al. 1966
- Bettelheim 1967
- Davids et al. 1968
- Weinstein 1969
- Alderton 1969
- Bender 1969
- Levy 1969
- Weiss and Weiss 1969

During the 1970s

- Hansen 1970
- Weiss and Burke 1970
- McConville and Purohit 1973
- Gamboa and Garrett 1974
- Lewis et al. 1975
- Davids and Salvatore 1976
- Kirby et al. 1977
- Mazuryk et al. 1978
- Stewart et al. 1978
- White et al. 1979

1980 through 1990

- Koret 1980
- Winsberg et al. 1980
- Schain et al. 1982
- Cohen-Sandler et al. 1982
- Oliver and Knight 1984
- Waldron and Nurias 1984
- Doherty et al. 1987
- Loff et al. 1987
- Parham et al. 1987
- Satterfield et al. 1987
- Asay et al. 1990
- Dalton et al. 1990
- Deblinger et al. 1990
- Gabel and Schindledecker 1990
- Kolko et al. 1990
- Thomsen 1990

Table 3–2. Efficacy studies (to date) that have examined outcome of short-term hospitalization

- Blinder et al. 1978
- Shafii et al. 1979
- Ney et al. 1984
- LaBarbera 1984
- Kazdin et al. 1987
- Dalton et al. 1990

higher intelligence is associated with favorable long-term results, while one produced equivocal findings and another showed that there was no correlation.

Diagnosis and symptom presentation have also been correlated with outcome. Seven studies have attempted to relate aggression and antisocial symptoms to outcome, nine have commented on psychosis, six on organic brain syndrome symptoms, two on autism, three on character-disorder symptoms, one on suicidal behavior, one on neurosis, and one on the relationship between phobic symptoms and follow-up findings. Except for psychosis, conduct disorder, and autism, each of which correlates with poor outcome, diagnosis seems to be a questionable predictor, at best. Little has been written about affective and anxiety disorders as predictors. Blotcky et al.'s caveat about the relationship between severe conduct and character pathology, on the one hand, and psychosis, on the other, is important. These commonly occurring overlaps obscure the validity of their relationship to outcome.

Symptom presentation might appear to be a more valid predictor, but the ability to quantify symptoms is an ongoing problem. One patient's aggressive behavior might pale in comparison with another's. Reliable measures are needed before comparison of patients among studies is possible.

Six studies have examined age and sex as possible predictive variables. Our own studies corroborate the general finding that very young hospitalized children have not done well at follow-up. Because of the lack of adequate controls, however, it is difficult to know whether age is a dependent variable related to the severity and early onset of serious psychopathology or an independent variable directly influencing follow-up status. The studies related to gender produce questionable, noncompelling results.

Any assessment of the contribution of family functioning to outcome must include the full range of parent, parenting, and family subvariables summarized by Blotcky et al. (1984):

1. Conceptualization of family functioning, including separation of genetic contributions from family-systems or interpersonal issues
2. The child's developmental level during the points of family crisis
3. The multitude of individual variables associated with each family member

Nevertheless, findings from Gabel and Shindledecker's (1990) recent study linking parent-family variables to poor patient outcome underscore the importance of this cluster of variables.

Ten studies have attempted to relate hospitalization and posthospitalization therapy variables to outcome. Teasing these variables apart so that they can be studied independently and interdependently requires the use of objective individual and family measures as well as multiple regressive statistical analyses. To date, only four studies have used such methodology. Kazdin and his colleagues (1987) prospectively investigated the combined effects of parent management training and cognitive-behavioral problem-solving skills training for 40 children with antisocial behaviors. At discharge and 1 year later the study group showed significantly less aggression and externalizing behavior at home and at school than did the control group. This investigation shed light not only on how to effectively treat this specific problem, but also on the type of follow-up research that is currently necessary in the field. Kolko and colleagues (1990) used a well-designed cognitive-behavioral group therapy program to impart appropriate social skills to conduct-disordered and hyperactive patients. When compared with boys exposed instead to a social activity group, the treatment groups showed significant improvement. Studies by Deblinger et al. (1990) and Satterfield et al. (1987) are reviewed in Chapter 9.

On the whole, the literature reinforces the previously held notion that it is the more seriously disturbed children who do worse at follow-up. Children with psychosis, serious organic pathology, autism with mental retardation, or antisocial symptoms, as well as those living with a parent with antisocial behavior, present with the most severe pathology 1 to 5 years following discharge. In addition, intelligent children and those who return to stable family environments tend to fare best at follow-up. These conclusions, however, say little about inpatient efficacy. Although large percentages of patients in numerous studies do well at follow-up, this research simply does not provide the evidence necessary to show how hospitalization affects their outcome.

We believe that more studies such as Kazdin et al.'s (1987) and Kolko et al.'s (1990) are needed to examine specific therapeutic approaches for specific clinical conditions, taking into account the relationship between child and interpersonal environment. When the data from these studies are compared with similarly collected data from other levels of care (e.g., residential facilities, day treatment, therapeutic foster homes), therapeutic efficacy will be much clearer.

In addition, several areas of inpatient practice require clarification by more global follow-up research. One relates to the controversy about whether patients with conduct disorders are best served on inpatient units, in residential facilities, or in community programs with good outpatient therapy. Prospective studies assigning patients randomly to each of these levels of care are necessary before a final determination can be made. Also, well-conceived prospective length-of-stay studies using multivariate analysis to correlate presenting symptoms, family functioning, hospital treatment approaches, length of stay, and longitudinal follow-up status, are essential to determine reasonable lengths of stay for specific patients' interpersonal and environmental problems. In addition, prospective studies assigning preschool patients with multiple problems randomly to either a psychiatric unit or a specialized foster care situation with appropriate psychiatric help should be undertaken before hospitalization for this age group becomes common.

Although we have thus far stressed efficacy studies, it would be remiss not to mention other types of research particularly suited for inpatient care. Riddle (1989) reviews four potential research areas: instrument development, the phenomenology of mixed disorders, clinical psychopharmacology, and neurochemical studies. Each of these offers a research opportunity without interfering with clinical evaluation and treatment.

Successfully chosen research projects are those that result naturally from questions raised in the course of clinical treatment. This process greatly increases treatment team interest and helps to overcome the typical obstacles (Riddle 1989). A qualified team member should be appointed to lead the research effort on the unit. Whether this responsibility includes everything from research design to data collection and analysis, or some part of the total approach, depends on many factors, including the availability of other research personnel. Because of the complexities of both sophisticated clinical work and sophisticated research, however, we do not think that the unit director, in most cases, has the time to do both equally well.

Confounding Issues

The nature of the research itself provides a major impediment to its inclusion in team activities. The logistical problems implicit in longitudinal studies, such as maintaining contact with discharged patients and engaging them in a research project after formal treatment has terminated, complicate matters. Devising a research design with appropriate control groups that will validly answer specific questions adds to the difficulty. The reliable measurement of patient behaviors and symptoms, as well as the complexities of family functioning, and environmental and treatment variables, pose additional problems. Pfeiffer and Strzelecki (1990) make useful recommendations for future investigations and suggest

1. A more complete delineation of the critical dimensions of inpatient treatment, including the various components of milieu therapy
2. A reexamination of what constitutes long-term success or positive adjustment
3. Employment of powerful statistical techniques and sophisticated designs
4. Expansion of an array of predictor variables, including social-interper-

sonal skills development, locus of control and attribution of responsibility, paternal presence within the home, and academic status, among others

The administrative design of a child inpatient unit can also be an obstacle. Unit research is a complex endeavor and demands coordination, cooperation, and uniformity. These requirements are very difficult to fulfill on units that operate without a strong unit director but have multiple teams who may use differing admission criteria and treatment approaches (see Chapter 15). Research concerns can impinge on clinical issues that require consistent and efficient decision making. Multiple decision-makers inherently make this task more difficult.

A third confounding issue is expense. While many sources of data are used in the course of usual unit functioning (e.g., rating scales, standardized psychological tests), the implementation of a well-designed program and the analysis of its results require the time and energy of professionals who must be reimbursed (Riddle 1989). Although indirect costs and expenses can often be provided (e.g., office space, computer time), most clinical settings do not pay individuals who are not directly involved in clinical care. Consequently, either clinical team members share research responsibilities—always a difficult proposition for busy team members—or professionals involved in research must be paid directly by the hospital or through grants.

Motivation and training can be major impediments. Many clinicians simply do not have the interest, while others do not recognize the importance of systematic study. Most child psychiatry fellowship training programs are exclusively clinically based. Often they do not provide the training necessary to understand which questions to ask, how to design a study to answer specific questions, how to implement the study and coordinate the collection of data, and how to analyze what has been collected. For research to be carried out on the inpatient service, the unit director must at least have some experience with research questions and must be able to support the research activities of other team members.

Research can sometimes interfere with clinical work. Inpatient protocols designed to study isolated, discrete therapy approaches make the use of other treatments impossible because these alternative therapies seriously confuse the interpretation of the study's results. Such research is acceptable if the treatment modality under study is designed to improve significantly the problematic child-environment fit (e.g., Kolko and colleagues' [1990] use of social-cognitive skills training groups for children with conduct disorders and attention-deficit disorder). In our opinion, studies investigating multimodal treatment approaches work best in an inpatient setting (e.g., Satterfield and colleagues' [1987] multimodal treatment study of predelinquent hyperactive boys), as they tend to approximate standard care more closely.

References

Alderton HR: A comparison of the follow-up status of Children's Aid Society wards and non-wards treated in a children's psychiatry hospital. Can Med Assoc J 100:1035–1042, 1969

Allerhand M, Weber R, Haug M: Adaptation and Adaptability: The Bellefaire Follow-up Study. New York, Child Welfare League of America, 1966

Asay T, Blotcky M, Dimperio T, et al: The Timberlawn Child Follow-up Study: intelligence and academic achievement as predictors of long-term post-hospital adjustment. Paper presented at the annual meeting of the American Academy of Child and Adolescent Psychiatry, Chicago, IL, October 1990

Bettelheim B: The Empty Fortress: Infantile Autism and the Birth of the Self. New York, Free Press, 1967

Bender L: A longitudinal study of schizophrenic children with autism. Hosp Community Psychiatry 20:230–237, 1969

Blinder BJ, Young WM, Fineman KR, et al: The children's psychiatric hospital unit in the community: I: concept and development. Am J Psychiatry 135:848–851, 1978

Blotcky MJ, Dimperio TL, Gossett JT: Follow-up of children treated in psychiatric hospitals: a review of studies. Am J Psychiatry 141:1499–1507, 1984

Cohen-Sandler R, Berman AL, King RA: A follow-up study of hospitalized suicidal children. J Am Acad Child Adolesc Psychiatry 21:398–403, 1982

Dalton R, Muller B, Forman M: The psychiatric hospitalization of children: an overview. Child Psychiatry Hum Dev 19:231–244, 1989

Dalton R, Bolding D, Forman M: The psychiatric hospitalization of preschool children: a follow-up study. Child Psychiatry Hum Dev 21:57–64, 1990

Davids A, Salvatore PD: Residential treatment of disturbed children and adequacy of their subsequent adjustment: a follow-up study. Am J Orthopsychiatry 46:62–73, 1976

Davids A, Ryan R, Salvatore PD: Effectiveness of residential treatment for psychotic and other disturbed children. Am J Orthopsychiatry 38:469–475, 1968

Deblinger E, McLeer SV, Henry D: Cognitive behavioral treatment for sexually abused children suffering from post-traumatic stress: preliminary findings. J Am Acad Child Adolesc Psychiatry 29:747–752, 1990

Doherty MB, Manderson M, Carter-Ake L: Time-limited hospitalization of children: a model and three-year outcome. Hosp Community Psychiatry 38:643–647, 1987

Gabel S, Shindledecker R: Parental substance abuse and suspected child abuse/maltreatment predict outcome in children's inpatient treatment. J Am Acad Child Adolesc Psychiatry 29:919–924, 1990

Gamboa AM Jr, Garrett JE: Re-education: a mental health service in an educational setting. Am J Orthopsychiatry 44:450–453, 1974

Hansen N: Cerebro-organic pathogenesis in 110 children followed up subsequent to admission to a child psychiatric department. Acta Psychiatr Scand 46:399–412, 1970

Johnson J, Rubin E: A school follow-up study of children discharged from a psychiatric hospital. Except Child 31:19–24, 1964

Kane RP, Chambers GS: Improvement—real or apparent? A seven year follow-up of children hospitalized and discharged from a residential setting. Am J Psychiatry 117:1023–1027, 1961

Kazdin AE, Esveldt-Dawson K, French NH, et al: Effects of parent management training and problem-solving skills training combined in the treatment of antisocial child behavior. J Am Acad Child Adolesc Psychiatry 26:416–424, 1987

Kirby TF, Wilson CT, Short MJ: A follow-up study of disturbed children treated in a Re-Ed program. Hosp Community Psychiatry 28:694–697, 1977

Kolko JD, Loar LL, Sturnick D: Inpatient social-cognitive skills training groups with conduct disordered and attention deficit disordered children. J Child Psychol Psychiatry 31:737–748, 1990

Koret S: Follow-up study on residential treatment of children, ages six through twelve. Journal of the National Association of Private Psychiatric Hospitals 11(3):43–47, 1980

LaBarbera J: Overcontrolled children and outcome of short-term psychiatric hospitalization. Child Psychiatry Hum Dev 15:21–33, 1984

Lawder D, Nordan R: What We Have Learned! A Report of the First Ten Years of the Astor Home, A Residential Treatment Center for Emotionally Disturbed Children. New York, Chartmakers, 1963

Levy EZ: Long-term follow-up of former inpatients at the Children's Hospital of the Menninger Clinic. Am J Psychiatry 125:1633–1639, 1969

Lewis SB, Barnhart FD, Gossett JT, et al: Follow-up of adolescents treated in a psychiatric hospital: operational solutions to some methodological problems of clinical research. Am J Orthopsychiatry 45:813–824, 1975

Loff CD, Trigg LJ, Cassels C: An evaluation of consumer satisfaction in a child psychiatric service: viewpoints of patients and parents. Am J Orthopsychiatry 57:132–134, 1987

Mazuryk GF, Barker P, Harasym L: Behavior therapy for autistic children: a study of acceptability and outcome. Child Psychiatry Hum Dev 9:119–125, 1978

McConville BJ, Purohit AP: Classifying confusion: a study of results of inpatient treatment in a multidisciplinary children's center. Am J Orthopsychiatry 43:411–417, 1973

Morris HH Jr, Escoll PJ, Wexler R: Aggressive behavior disorders of childhood: a follow-up study. Am J Psychiatry 112:991–997, 1956

Ney PG, Mulvihill D, Hanna R: The effectiveness of child psychiatry inpatient care. Can J Psychiatry 29(2):26–30, 1984

Oliver J, Knight D: An evaluation of an inpatient psychiatric unit for children. Child: Care, Health, and Development 10:141–155, 1984

Östman O: Psychiatric hospital care of children and adolescents in Sweden. Acta Psychiatr Scand 77:567–574, 1988

Parham C, Reid L, Harmmer R: A long-range follow-up study of former inpatients at a children's psychiatric hospital. Child Psychiatry Hum Dev 17:199–209, 1987

Pfeiffer SI, Strzelecki SC: Inpatient psychiatric treatment of children and adolescents: a review of outcome studies. J Am Acad Child Adolesc Psychiatry 29:847–853, 1990

Riddle MA: Research on a children's psychiatric inpatient service. J Am Acad Child Adolesc Psychiatry 28:42–46, 1989

Rosenthal FM, Pinsky GD: Follow-up method in child guidance work: a report on the method of follow-up used at the Child Guidance Home. Am J Orthopsychiatry 6:609–615, 1936

Satterfield JH, Satterfield BT, Schell AM: Therapeutic interventions to prevent delinquency in hyperactive boys. J Am Acad Child Adolesc Psychiatry 26:56–64, 1987

Schain RJ, Gardella D, Pon J: Five-year outcome of children admitted to a state mental hospital. Hosp Community Psychiatry 33:847–848, 1982

Shafii M, McCue A, Ice JF, et al: The development of an acute short-term inpatient child psychiatric setting: a pediatric-psychiatric model. Am J Psychiatry 136:427–429, 1979

Stewart MA, Adams CC, Meardon JK: Unsocialized aggressive boys: a follow-up study. J Clin Psychiatry 39:797–799, 1978

Thomsen P: The prognosis in early adulthood of child psychiatric patients: a case register study in Denmark. Acta Psychiatr Scand 81:89–93, 1990

Waldron J, Nurias P: Assessment of behavioral change in a child psychiatric inpatient program. Child Psychiatry Hum Dev 15:121–132, 1984

Weinstein L: Re-Ed schools for emotionally disturbed children: effectiveness as viewed by referring agencies, parents, and teachers. Except Child 35:703–711, 1969

Weiss M, Burke A: A 5- to 10-year follow-up of hospitalized school phobic children and adolescents. Am J Orthopsychiatry 40:672–676, 1970

Weiss V, Weiss S: Follow-up Study of Children Released From Residential Treatment Centers. New Orleans, LA, Jewish Children's Home Service, 1969

White T, Benn R, Gross D, et al: Assessing the need for follow-up: the relationship of prognosis to posthospitalization adjustment. Child Psychiatry Hum Dev 10:91–102, 1979

Winsberg BG, Bialer I, Kupietz S, et al: Home vs hospital care of children with behavior disorders: a controlled investigation. Arch Gen Psychiatry 37:413–418, 1980

Zick FT: Outcome of intramural psychotherapy of children. Smith College Studies in Social Work 14:127–132, 1943

Chapter 4

Indications for Admission

Indications for the admission of children to psychiatric units are the product of an interplay among patient, family, environmental, and treatment factors. The needs of the child and family, as well as the community's ability to meet those needs, serve as specific determinants in individual cases. Indirectly, however, the decision for each hospitalization must also be based on potential advantages and disadvantages.

Advantages

Harper's (1989) review of the possible advantages of hospitalization underscores what this therapeutic approach selectively offers. This approach provides clinicians a chance to make accurate diagnostic assessments as they observe the child at work and at play within a controlled environment. It also enables them to see how the child reacts to family, peers, and professionals. Clinicians observe the functioning of the family as it turns the care of the child over to unit workers. Hospitalization provides a major strategic opportunity for long-term treatment planning as well as an excellent setting for intensive therapy. Furthermore, the controlled environment ensures safety and security as well as the provision of nurturance.

Disadvantages

Possible disadvantages must also be considered. The disruption of the child's family and community relationships and the expense of hospitalization are potentially the most negative effects. In addition, the hospitalization process can reinforce parental denial or guilt and leave the patient's siblings with confused and distorted perceptions. The removal of the child from the continuum of the education system and the potential for unresolved transference and dependency attachments to the hospital must also be considered. Predictable obnoxious stigmata and labeling can result (Stone 1979). Furthermore, the child's lack of understanding regarding the reasons for hospitalization can undermine the treatment process and negatively contribute to the outcome (Szajnberg and Weiner 1989). Of course, hospitalizations occurring for inappropriate reasons frequently lead to negative feelings that have long-term consequences for the patient and family.

Criteria

Admission criteria have evolved considerably through the years and reflect changes within the larger field of child mental health. Bradley (1949) believed that psychiatric hospitalization should be considered as an appropriate treatment when the child's need for an accepting environment could not otherwise be provided. This environment-dependent criterion, however, reflected the paucity of out-of-home placement alternatives during the 1930s and 1940s.

Dettelbach's (1955) reduction of admission criteria into quantitative (aggressive and destructive behaviors), qualitative (specific diagnoses), and parental factors (the inability to adequately contain, or the covert encouragement of, destructive behaviors) corresponded with the increased sophistication of data collection and organization within child psychiatry and psychology. She was among the first to call for hospital or residential placement when the severity of patient problems precluded treatment in less restrictive settings.

From the 1940s to the 1970s, concurrent with the application of psychodynamics to inpatient care, indications changed accordingly. Stone (1979) divided patient variables into intrapsychic, developmental, and environmental categories. Specific examples included disturbances in object relations regarding the capacity for attachment, unrealistic self-image, and inappropriate affective responses, among others. Although an improvement over previously presented indicators, these categories appear vague and imprecise by today's standards.

During the 1980s, with the burgeoning growth of inpatient units and the increased sophistication of hospital therapeutic interventions, admission criteria further evolved. The almost exclusive emphasis that had been placed on patient variables was supplanted by a set of general guidelines based on multiple factors.

Hersov and Bentovim (1985, p. 767) have summarized currently accepted criteria for admission:

1. Where thought behaviour and affective display are so severely irrational and bizarre that out-patient treatment is impossible, or where the child may be a danger to himself [or herself] or to others.
2. Where socially unacceptable behaviour arises from a degree of psychiatric disorder that is unaffected by ordinary social measures of removal from home or outpatient treatment.
3. Where a complex psychiatric problem requires skilled observation integrated with assessment and treatment that must be continuous and of an intensity not possible on an outpatient basis.
4. Where the family interaction is so distorted that life at home leads to continuing or progressive interference with the child's development and progress. In this situation the child may need a controlled therapeutic environment to provide healthier life experiences and relationships.
5. For specific assessment and treatment such as a double-blind controlled trial of medication which cannot be carried out as an out-patient; [or] for stabilization of anti-epileptic medication which may be affecting cognitive and behavioral function; . . .
6. To treat a life-threatening illness such as anorexia nervosa, intractable asthma or suicidal depressive disorder.

To make a sensible judgment the clinician must consider the patient's symptoms and diagnostic clusters in conjunction with the family's ability to manage these behaviors, as well as the community's ability to assist the family in containing and treating the problems and to provide effective alternatives to hospitalization. While it is difficult to specify which particular symptom patterns and behaviors are invariably suitable for hospital treatment, some are obviously more suitable than others. Among those generally thought to be appropriate are psychotic symptoms secondary to schizophrenia, affective disorder, and pervasive developmental disorder; self-destructive behavior seen in patients with borderline personality traits, organic personality disorder, and eating disorders; and suicidal behavior. These symptoms more often than not require the skilled psychiatric, medical, and nursing care offered on inpatient units.

Several other behavioral and diagnostic clusters often, but not invariably, require hospitalization. Separation-anxiety disorder associated with school phobia that has not responded to outpatient management and therapy is appropriate for inpatient treatment. Dangerously aggressive and disruptive behavior seen in children with conduct disorder requires inpatient hospitalization when less restrictive care either has been ineffective or is unavailable. Nonpsychotic patients with serious depression who require a thorough diagnostic evaluation, treatment planning, and skilled medical and nursing care are appropriate for inpatient care. Tourette's syndrome, functional encopresis, and childhood substance abuse disorders might also require inpatient treatment for purposes of diagnostic assessment and treatment planning when less restrictive options have proven ineffective. Destructive and overly disruptive behaviors secondary to organic personality disorder or other character disorders, as well as acute anxiety, dysphoria, and behavioral acting out related to posttraumatic stress disorder, might also be suitable.

Family interactional patterns that promote psychological or physical illness or substantially impede normal development often appropriately lead to placement outside of the home. Hospitalization should be chosen when the child's own behavior warrants it and when less restrictive settings are not able to manage interference from the family.

Uncomplicated bereavement, mental retardation, functional enuresis, stereotypic movement disorders, overanxious disorder, and avoidant disorder are not, in and of themselves, appropriate for admission. Furthermore, symptoms and behaviors that are secondary to uncomplicated oppositional disorder and uncomplicated attention-deficit disorder rarely require hospitalization.

The results of a recent clinical study show that clinicians are, by and large, using these indicators to facilitate decision making (Mabe et al. 1990). In an examination of the most important criteria actually used to determine the need for inpatient care, clinical directors of public and private units chose severity of symptoms, ineffectiveness of outpatient treatment, medical complications, and the family's ability to safely contain the child as the most frequent indicators for admission. Diagnosis, though generally seen as important by third-party payers, was chosen seventh overall among 12 possibilities. Nevertheless, Rogeness et al.'s (1988) recent review of diagnoses applied to 763 consecutive admissions (some with multiple diagnoses), as shown in Table 4–1, is very consistent with our experience on our university and state hospital units.

Table 4–1. Diagnoses applied to consecutive admissions on an inpatient unit ($N = 763$)

Diagnosis	Percentage of sample having diagnosis
Conduct disorder	50
Dysthymia	25
Narcissistic and borderline personality disorders	20
Overanxious and avoidant disorders	11
Major depression	10
Schizophrenia	7

Source. Data adapted from Rogeness et al. 1988.

Long-Term Hospitalization

As discussed in Chapter 2, long-term hospitalization results from an unfortunate combination of patient, family, and community variables. One clear preadmission indication involves individuals with serious psychopathology who have previously been unsuccessfully treated in less restrictive settings, including short-term hospitalization. In addition, there are patients whose pathology and aggressive behavior are so pervasive and intractable (e.g., some cases of organic personality disorder, schizophrenia, and severe character pathology) that skilled clinicians, knowing the specific patient and available community resources, might correctly opt for extensive hospitalization.

While there might well be other examples that meet the criteria for planned, long-term hospitalization and that do not easily fit into one of these categories, we think that generally the indications are limited. Furthermore, even when valid, patients admitted for long-term hospitalization ought to be reviewed regularly by the treatment team for possible movement to a less restrictive setting.

Unplanned Admissions

Unplanned admissions provide obvious problems for the patient, family, and treatment team. The suddenness of the move from home to the hospital can appear to the patient to be an impulsive response by caregivers and doctors, making subsequent alliance building and the development of trust more difficult. Also, parents may feel that they have been coerced by the admitting psychiatrist without having their fears and resistances adequately addressed. In such circumstances, they may never effectively join the treatment process. Siblings are also vulnerable. They are more likely to interpret an emergency admission of a brother or sister as a personal threat. Furthermore, without adequate preparation, treatment planning itself is delayed until the patient is actually hospitalized. This delay seriously impedes the early development of an effective therapeutic program and often increases the eventual length of stay. In short, admissions should be planned in advance whenever possible to give the family, patient, siblings, and treatment team members time to adequately prepare.

Serious suicidal thoughts and actions, seriously self-destructive actions, and serious physical violence that cannot otherwise be contained are indications for emergency hospitalization. Acutely psychotic children who become destructive might well require an unplanned admission, whereas nondestructive acutely psychotic patients might not. Depressed children who express the wish to die but are willing to engage in the treatment process might not be candidates for emergency inpatient treatment, whereas those who will not be engaged, or who have shown by their actions a serious intent to harm themselves, are certainly candidates. A patient whose outwardly directed aggression has suddenly become uncontrollable is a candidate if the behavior is secondary to a psychiatric disorder. Serious physical or sexual abuse noted during an emergency room or clinic visit in a child who cannot be reasonably managed on a pediatric unit might require an unplanned psychiatric admission. However, oppositional struggles between children and parents, school phobia, intermittent aggression or thoughts of aggression, and uncomplicated psychotic behavior are not indications for unplanned admissions.

Confounding Issues

Despite the increased specificity of hospitalization criteria, there are several issues that confound the decision-making process. Among them is the fact that the previously mentioned criteria have been based on clinicians' experiences with inpatient settings and outpatient therapy. The spectrum of services developed during the past several decades (residential facilities, group homes, therapeutic foster care, and day-treatment settings) to provide an alternative to hospitalization when outpatient care has proven ineffective has not yet been adequately factored into the equation. In fact, no research exists comparing efficacy of treatment among these levels of care (Goldfine et al. 1985). Although Winsberg and colleagues (1980) attempted a prospective study to measure the effectiveness of outpatient versus inpatient care, problems with methodology and inter-rater reliability significantly confused possible meaningful conclusions. In short, the decision regarding hospitalization ultimately rests on the clinician's judgment of how effective each level of care within the community has been with specific diagnostic entities and symptom patterns. The chosen level of care should be the least restrictive, most efficient approach possible to effectively treat the patient and family problems.

The decision-making process is further complicated within the private sector by contemporary economic and medical practice issues. The rapid growth of psychiatric for-profit hospitals and school-age units during the 1970s and 1980s (Thompson et al. 1982) has led to stiff competition and aggressive marketing practices that, in turn, have contributed to a greatly increased number of admissions. Psychiatrists employed or given inducements by for-profit hospitals are often pressured in subtle and not-so-subtle ways to maintain a maximal census and, thus, to increase profits (Eisenberg 1984). Such pressure can lead to psychiatric practice changes not fully acknowledged by the physician; a bias toward inpatient hospitalization can develop. Furthermore, standard practices by third-party payers encourage admissions by offering greater reimbursement for inpatient care than for outpatient treatment.

University departments also place demands on faculty to maintain a maximal census as financial difficulties secondary to federal cutbacks during the 1980s have fueled a search for additional revenue for funding support for residents and faculty. This has in turn contributed to an expansion of inpatient services within university hospitals. In addition, child psychiatry training programs depend on inpatient services for gathering clinical case material for student and resident training (Dalton and Forman 1987).

There are pressures contributing to unnecessary, unplanned admissions in the public sector. Because unit directors often do not have control over the admissions process, but must instead offer available beds to children deemed appropriate by clinicians in local mental health centers, patients are often sent to the hospital to be directly admitted. Sometimes their symptoms meet the necessary criteria, but sometimes they do not.

Judicial commitments can lead to unplanned admissions in both the public and the private sectors. Patients are typically taken from the courtroom to the hospital, offering no time for a reasonable transition. While such patients are usually difficult to treat, at best, the suddenness of the hospitalization can also certainly contribute to a subsequent negative therapeutic response.

Unplanned admissions in the private sector are also common. With current marketing practices, corporate hospitals frequently advertise free evaluations 24 hours per day for children with problematic behavior. Disruptive children are often seen by these emergency evaluation teams whose main purposes are to determine whether the presenting complaints are suitable for hospitalization and the family's ability to pay for the services. Evaluation personnel are not particularly interested in determining whether less restrictive measures would be effective. These children are frequently admitted following the evaluation and are assigned to the next physician on the call list.

Adhering to the particular clinical guidelines we have described can help ensure that the decision to hospitalize a particular child is in the patient's best interest. Clinicians should be aware of the conscious and unconscious pressures that they face to put the institution's needs (and their own) before the patient's. If the clinician is unsure about the most effective treatment level to offer for a particular constellation of problems, a less restrictive setting should be chosen first. If that level fails, then hospitalization would be more readily considered. Of course, asking a colleague for a second opinion is always an appropriate option.

Admissions Process

The handling of the admissions process is very important in establishing trust and in engaging the patient and family in the treatment process. Several issues must be anticipated and addressed prior to the actual admission (American Academy of Child and Adolescent Psychiatry 1990). The reason inpatient treatment is recommended and how it will help the patient, as well as possible treatment alternatives to inpatient treatment, should be discussed with the family. The qualifications and training of the clinicians involved and the unit's suitability for school-age children are explicitly described to the family. Components of inpatient treatment as well as the responsibilities of the treatment team members, including the child psychiatrist, should be elaborated. Parent involvement in the hospitalization decision-making processes and in preliminary posthospitalization treatment plans is reviewed.

Once clinical suitability for hospitalization is determined, and the parents have decided that inpatient treatment is necessary for substantive change, financial matters are discussed. Along with an estimated length of stay, the clinician should clearly explain potential hospital costs and doctor's fees. The parents then meet with business office representatives to ultimately determine the economic feasibility of admission. The clinician and family discuss what will happen if the family can no longer afford hospitalization that the patient continues to require. (See Chapter 15 for a discussion of clinician intervention with hospital administrators for patients and families with limited insurance coverage.)

The admissions process itself should begin prior to the first day of hospitalization; the treatment team should have made their evaluation (see Chapter 5) and already begun to establish an alliance with the patient and family, who may have toured the unit during a previous outpatient visit. Other unit patients and staff have been prepared for the patient's admission. These preparations, which differentiate planned from unplanned admissions, can have a major effect on the treatment process in general.

On the day of admission, the clinician meets the family and patient to discuss what will happen during the process, to answer questions, and to deal with anxieties. The clinician goes with the family to the unit, introduces the patients and staff to the new patient and family, and helps the patient and family say good-bye to each other. Patients are given time to collect themselves and then are involved in the milieu and unit process.

Nurses explain unit rules to the patient. Nursing staff members go through personal belongings while one staff member integrates the patient into the milieu and begins to develop an alliance. An explanation is given to the parents about the unit routine, including phone calls, visits, and passes. The nurses procure information from the parents regarding the patient's living habits, self-help skills, fears, and other attributes important to the milieu. The parents sign necessary permissions at this time.

The transition from home to the hospital can be very traumatic. All staff members must be sensitive to patient and family anxieties and must approach them supportively. A thoughtful admissions process can positively affect the overall implementation of the treatment plan.

References

American Academy of Child and Adolescent Psychiatry: Facts for Families, No 32. Washington, DC, American Academy of Child and Adolescent Psychiatry, January 1990

Bradley C: Indications for residential treatment of children with severe neuropsychiatric problems. Am J Orthopsychiatry 19:427–431, 1949

Dalton R, Forman MA: Conflicts of interest associated with the psychiatric hospitalization of children. Am J Orthopsychiatry 57:12–14, 1987

Dettelbach MH: The role of residential treatment for children: criteria for agency referral of a child to a residential treatment center. Am J Orthopsychiatry 25:669–674, 1955

Eisenberg L: The case against for-profit hospitals. Hosp Community Psychiatry 35:1009–1013, 1984

Goldfine PE, Heath GA, Hardesty VA, et al: Alternatives to psychiatric hospitalization for children. Psychiatr Clin North Am 8:527–535, 1985

Harper GT: Focal inpatient treatment planning. J Am Acad Child Adolesc Psychiatry 28:31–37, 1989

Hersov L, Bentovim A: In-patient and day-hospital units, in Child and Adolescent Psychiatry: Modern Approaches, 2nd Edition. Edited by Rutter M, Hersov L. Oxford, UK, Blackwell Scientific, 1985, pp 766–779

Mabe P, Riley W, Sunde E: Survey of admission policies for child and adolescent inpatient services: a national sample. Child Psychiatry Hum Dev 20:99–111, 1990

Rogeness GA, Hoppe SK, Macedo CA, et al: Psychopathology in hospitalized, adopted children. J Am Acad Child Adolesc Psychiatry 27:628–631, 1988

Stone LA: Residential treatment, in Basic Handbook of Child Psychiatry, Vol 3: Therapeutic Interventions. Edited by Harrison SI (JD Noshpitz, Editor-in-Chief). New York, Basic Books, 1979, pp 231–262

Szajnberg N, Weiner A: Children's conceptualization of their own psychiatric illness and hospitalization. Child Psychiatry Hum Dev 20:87–97, 1989

Thompson JW, Bass RD, Witkin MJ: Fifty years of psychiatric services: 1940–1990. Hosp Community Psychiatry 33:711–717, 1982

Winsberg BG, Bialer I, Kupietz S, et al: Home vs hospital care of children with behavior disorders: a controlled investigation. Arch Gen Psychiatry 37:413–418, 1980

Chapter 5

Evaluation

The inpatient evaluation involves not only the diagnostic assessment of the patient and family but also the review and monitoring of the entire therapeutic process. There are six main purposes for the psychiatric inpatient evaluation (Table 5–1):

1. To discern the patient's developmental levels, including an assessment of the child's intellectual, social, and psychological functioning, as well as the family's level of functioning.
2. To elucidate the presence and type of psychopathology in the patient, within the family, and in family members, including a thorough evaluation of problems in the mis-fit between child and interpersonal environment (see Chapter 2). Both dynamic formulations and specific diagnoses are proffered.
3. To assess whether the patient is appropriate for hospitalization. Curiously, this might logically be presumed to be the first purpose, but it clinically follows purposes 1 and 2 above. If the child does not require hospitalization, an assessment of the level of care necessary for amelioration of the problems is indicated.
4. To discern whether there are specific patient symptoms that require special management in the milieu. Evaluation and subsequent treatment planning for possible aggression (psychotic or nonpsychotic), sexual acting out, fire setting, runaway behavior, suicidal behavior, encopresis, enuresis, psychotic aggression, masochistic behavior (in patients with borderline personality traits), oppositionalism, and profound anxiety should be undertaken as soon as possible (see Chapter 13). Also, the patient's self-help and social skills must be assessed.
5. To help determine the specific treatment goals for each inpatient's stay. This formulation depends not only on a thorough assessment of the patient and family but also on therapeutic resources available in the community.

6. To evaluate, on an ongoing basis, the patient's response to the treatment process. This is important not only because it clarifies the effectiveness of the process, but also because it provides additional diagnostic information about the patient and family as the hospitalization proceeds.

The evaluation process is discussed in detail below and is summarized in Table 5–2.

Before Hospitalization

Except in the event of unplanned or emergency admissions, the evaluation process begins prior to hospitalization. Although the prehospitalization evaluation process involves a total assessment of the patient and family, it is most concerned with determining patient suitability for admission. The two main components of this process are *data gathering* and *team conferences.* Data-gathering procedures include the psychiatric examination, psychological testing, family evaluation, clinical rating scales, individual psychiatric examinations of family members when necessary, a review of reports from previous diagnostic and therapeutic efforts, and a review of the patient's social history and school reports, among others. Subsequent team conferences are designed to organize the collected data, to discuss patient and family psychological status, and ultimately to determine suitability for hospitalization. Following that, initial treatment planning determines overall long-term treatment goals as well as specific goals for the patient's hospitalization, the inpatient treatment components necessary to achieve hospitalization goals, preliminary discharge criteria, and posthospitalization treatment components required to satisfy long-term goals (see Chapter 6).

Table 5–1. Main purposes for the psychiatric inpatient evaluation (in temporal order)

1. To discern the patient's developmental levels
2. To elucidate the presence and type of psychopathology in the patient, within the family, and in family members
3. To assess whether the patient is appropriate for hospitalization
4. To discern whether there are specific patient symptoms that require special management in the milieu
5. To help determine the specific treatment goals for each inpatient's stay
6. To evaluate, on an ongoing basis, the patient's response to the treatment process

Marsden and colleagues' (1977) review of patient selection procedures has statistically correlated the conference and data-gathering activities with the subsequent duration of hospitalization as well as with the percentage of referrals rejected. The authors noted a wide discrepancy among the 39 institutions questioned and concluded that thorough preadmission assessments, including family evaluations and the review of previous work-ups, are in the patient's best interest.

Intake

The first data-gathering procedure is usually an intake interview with parents or guardians to determine the chief complaint and related information. Thorough developmental, medical, educational, and social histories are obtained. A family history of psychiatric and physical illnesses is sought, and current environmental and stress-related events are discussed.

Rating Scales

During the past decade, rating scales have been developed both to identify children in the community with symptom and behavior clusters suggestive of specific diagnostic entities and to record how many symptoms are indicative of a specific illness a particular child may be experiencing.

Although there are several scales available in outpatient settings, only the revised Child Behavior Checklist (CBCL) (Achenbach and Edelbrock 1983) has established norms for school-age inpatients (Jones et al. 1988). Because of its empirically derived scales, the abundance of objective information it provides about several diagnostic clusters, its versions for children, parents, teachers, and direct caregivers, as well as its previously defined inpatient norms, the CBCL is by far the most useful scale. Other

Table 5–2. The inpatient evaluation process

Before hospitalization
- Intake
- Rating scales
- Psychiatric examination
- Structured interviews
- Psychological tests
- Family evaluations and interviews
- Teacher/principal interviews
- Review of previous evaluations

Early part of hospitalization
- Physical examination
- Laboratory tests
- Advanced technologies
- Dexamethasone suppression test
- Neurological consultation
- Pediatric subspecialty consultations

Later part of hospitalization
- Rating scales for ongoing reevaluation
- Clinical data on patient and family response to treatment

scales are used to assess hyperactivity (Conners 1973), depression (Costello and Angold 1988; Kovacs 1981; Poznanski et al. 1979), social skills (Matson et al. 1983), anxiety disorders (Gittelman 1985; Spielberger 1973), eating disorders (Halmi et al. 1981), obsessive-compulsive disorder (Berg et al. 1985), pharmacotherapy side effects (Fann et al. 1980), and autism (Schopler et al. 1985).

The use of rating scales, particularly the CBCL, facilitates the assessment process. In addition to the efficiency and cost effectiveness of these scales, several advantages accrue from their use, including the collection of objective data incorporating direct observations (Kolko 1988). The importance of these scales for research is obvious. The usefulness of rating scales for clinical work depends on the treatment team's ability to collect, analyze, and therapeutically respond to the data. In our experience rating scales can provide substantial help in identifying underlying depression and anxiety in children with very obstreperous behavior. The CBCL aggression subscale can predict future inpatient aggression in some school-age patients (Garrison et al. 1990). McLeer et al. (1988) have demonstrated the superiority of the CBCL in evaluating posttraumatic stress disorder in sexually abused patients when compared with other rating scales.

Psychiatric Examination

The psychiatric examination of the child is the most important evaluation procedure (Cox and Rutter 1985). It is helpful to start with an open-ended approach to gauge the child's unconscious issues, underlying developmental level, and methods of handling needs during usual situations and during times of stress. Eliciting projective data can be facilitated by the use of mutual story telling and play therapy techniques as well as by asking for specific wishes, dreams, and stories. As the exam proceeds, the clinician asks specific questions about a range of issues designed to detail patient perceptions about symptoms and behaviors. The patient's strengths and assets are fully assessed. Throughout, the examiner should present with a sympathetic, reflective, encouraging, and understanding demeanor. Empathy and warmth are important, but they should not lead to an overly intrusive or overly intimate approach with the patient.

Structured Interviews

Structured psychiatric examinations, such as the Schedule for Affective Disorders and Schizophrenia for School-Age Children (Kiddie-SADS) (Puig-Antich and Chambers 1978), the Child Assessment Schedule (Hodges et al. 1982), the Diagnostic Interview for Children and Adolescents (DICA) (Herjanic and Reich 1982), and the Diagnostic Interview Schedule for Children (A. Costello, C. Edelbrock, M. Dulean, et al., unpublished manuscript, 1984) are often used for research purposes. Because they are cumbersome and insensitive to DSM Axis II traits, they currently play a limited role in standard hospital clinical evaluations. However, they do provide reliable information about symptom and diagnostic clusters and, thus, can significantly contribute to the evaluation process. Considering both the scope of the data provided and the ease of administration, the DICA should be chosen first, in our opinion.

Psychological Tests

The use of psychological testing in determining patient suitability for admission as well as specific psychological weaknesses and attributes is limited. However, data obtained from intelligence tests and the analysis of their subscales provide very useful material about the patient's intellectual level and cognitive abilities as well as potential neurological and organically based difficulties. Understanding what the subscales contribute to the assessment of left-brain and right-brain functioning can be very important in evaluating the patient's ability to correctly perceive and interpret internal and environmental events. Projective psychological tests, though often used, offer little diagnostically (Gittelman 1980) and are of very limited use in determining suitability for admission. They can be useful, however, during hospitalization in helping to determine whether a patient has an underlying disintegrative ego deficit substantially contributing to the development and maintenance of symptomatic behaviors.

Family Evaluations

Parent and family evaluations are critical in developing an understanding of the patient's relatedness within the environment. There are both short-term and long-term goals for these evaluations. The short-term aims involve the collection of those data that can be gathered in one or two sessions and that are necessary for the establishment and implementation of the initial treatment plan. These include familial genetic proclivities to psychiatric disorders, major individual psychopathology in family members, serious and dangerous acting out by family members, and family willingness to participate in the treatment process. Longer-term goals, which might require the entire hospitalization to elucidate, include the understanding of individual roles within the family, the rigidity with which these roles are maintained, how the family resolves conflict, individual identity and ego autonomy issues within the family, and subtle manipulations and defense mechanisms used to maintain the family structure and individual and family self-esteem (Scharff 1989). In essence, the evaluation process continues throughout hospitalization, constantly leading to the modification of treatment goals and approaches as new information becomes available.

The use of rating scales to assess family functioning has not developed as quickly as the use of these scales for individual functioning, and none has standardized norms for inpatient work. The Family Environment Scale (Moos and Moos 1981) is very useful for outpatient work. However, because each family member must answer written questions, its potential with younger children is limited. The modified Camberwell Family Interview for Children (CFI-C), a semistructured interview designed to discern the impact of the child's behavior on the family, is useful, although its administration is fairly cumbersome (Asarnow et al. 1987).

Other Data

Collecting and evaluating data from nonfamily members can also be very important. After permission is obtained, it is useful to talk with the patient's teacher, principal, or school counselor for information about behavior in the classroom, behavior with significant adults outside of the home, peer relationships, adaptive functioning during times of stress, and information regarding academic performance. The teacher version of the CBCL can provide additional information (Achenbach and Edelbrock 1983). The clinician should also speak with other adults with whom the patient spends time (e.g., grandparents) for their perspectives. Previous reports from social agencies and mental health professionals should also be reviewed.

Early Part of Hospitalization

Physical Examination

Evaluations during the early part of hospitalization start with a review of systems and physical examination of the child, with special emphasis paid to the neurological exam.

Laboratory Tests

The laboratory portion of the workup usually includes a complete blood count with differential, a urinalysis, and a chemistry panel with an electrolyte profile. An electrocardiogram is ordered if there is a family history of depression or separation anxiety and tricyclic antidepressant medications are being considered. Other procedures (e.g., thyroid panel, diagnostic tests specific for other organic illnesses) are ordered when indicated by patient symptoms or family history, or when baseline data prior to medication usage are needed (see Chapter 8). Although Ricciuti and colleagues (1987) have noted that routine laboratory tests are of little clinical value on child inpatient units in that they rarely yield productive results, we nevertheless procure them because, in conjunction with the physical exam, they have been useful in identifying clinical needs in previously neglected and abused children currently in the custody of the state.

Advanced Technologies

New, advanced technologies currently used in adult psychiatry and other medical fields—for example, CAT scans and magnetic resonance imaging (MRI); chromosomal analysis; biochemical assessment of neuroendocrine, neurotransmitter, and medication levels in blood or urine; refined neuropsychiatric assessments—are increasingly employed for school-age inpatient diagnostic purposes. Woolston and Riddle's (1990) study suggests that these technologies provide a moderately positive yield, considering cost, and that they will be increasingly used in the future. Our experience has been that genetic and chromosomal studies and antidepressant blood levels are very helpful.

Dexamethasone Suppression Test

Although the dexamethasone suppression test (DST) can be useful in identifying depression, it generally remains a research tool with child psychiatric inpatients. In a recent study by Weller et al. (1990), depressed inpatients were nonsuppressors (72%) significantly more often than were depressed outpatients (50%), psychiatric control subjects (22%), or normal control subjects (6%).

Neurological Consultation

A neurological consultation is sought when there are positive neurological findings on the physical exam or when there is a history suggestive of neurological problems or seizures. Furthermore, a significant difference between verbal and performance intelligence as measured on the subscales of intelligence tests, as well as sudden behavioral changes without obvious environmental precipitants, is a reason for a pediatric neurological consultation. All neurological consultations should be accompanied by a sleep-deprived electroencephalogram.

We have consulted pediatric neurology 10 times for our last 50 university unit patients. Other specialties have been less frequently consulted: general pediatrics has been consulted 9 times, and pediatric cardiology, gastroenterology, pulmonary medicine, and gynecology each has been consulted on 3 occasions. Although there are no reliable confirmatory data, we suspect that child inpatient units within general hospitals or in children's hospitals are more likely to treat children with concurrent pediatric illnesses (e.g., cystic fibrosis, asthma, chronic heart disease) and thus are likely to consult other subspecialists more often than are units in free-standing psychiatric hospitals.

Finally, during the early part of hospitalization, it is important to consider follow-up treatment options available in the community. Specifically, the appropriateness of each level of care in attuning the previously described fit is considered. This may be a relatively simple process for clinicians who are familiar with the services offered within their communities.

Later Part of Hospitalization

As hospitalization proceeds, so does the evaluation process. The continual assessment of the child's relationship to the milieu, peers, and staff members, as well as within the therapies, offers very important information about the patient's sense of self, psychopathology, strengths, and progress. As previously stated, one of the major advantages of hospitalization is the opportunity for this type of thorough, ongoing assessment. The use of weekly rating scales can facilitate this endeavor. Choosing the most useful and efficient rating scale is not easy. Just as we have previously described for general scales, few consecutively used rating scales have been standardized for inpatient settings (Orvaschel and Walsh 1984), and, among those that have, utility is limited because of questionable reliability and validity (Raskin 1982). However, Kolko's (1988) examination of the factor structure, reliability, and validity of the Child Behavior Rating Form (CBRF) derived from the CBCL (Achenbach and Edelbrook 1983) is quite encouraging. It provides useful information about symptom variability as well as response to behavioral and pharmacological therapy. It reflects highly visible, high-frequency behaviors, thus facilitating the evaluation of the severity of the child's psychopathology. Although, as Kolko points out, its sensitivity to treatment outcome and its reliability across raters, time, and diagnostic groups are yet to be fully determined, it is more promising than any of the previously designed scales.

The Ward Atmosphere Scale (Moos 1974) has been shown to be useful in evaluating treatment milieus (Feist et al. 1985). It helps staff evaluate the unit holding environment on an ongoing basis (see Chapter 12).

Confounding Issues

The same issues that create the previously discussed conflicts of interest (see Chapter 4) can also contribute to inadequate evaluations. The 24-hour emergency teams mentioned in Chapter 4 often admit patients after very limited assessments. Unplanned admissions may result in a less thorough diagnostic and assessment process. Delaying diagnostic evaluations until after the patient has been admitted to the hospital can lead to premature treatment planning, especially when the length of hospitalization is shortened because of financial limitations. Furthermore, clinicians with too many inpatients, and thus not enough time, often cut corners by hastening evaluations. Other issues confounding the process include poor coordination among team members and misinterpretation of the generated data.

The consistent use of rating scales is often overlooked because they involve a time-consuming process: the data must be collated, reviewed, and understood by the treatment team. The collection and analysis of the data for clinical purposes requires a structured, authority-oriented team and unit administrative approach (see Chapter 15). It also requires large amounts of time from at least one team member. The choice to use unit resources in this manner depends on the unit's clinical and research goals as well as on the team members' confidence in and experience with this approach to evaluation.

Conversely, over-reliance on or exclusive usage of rating scales can also be a problem. Rating scales do not provide information about patient and family motivation for particular actions and behaviors. In short, they do not tell the examiner about patients' perceptions of why they have said or done specific things. That information is as important as discerning the presence and quantity of specific behaviors and symptom clusters, and can be obtained only through ongoing, open-ended assessment.

References

Achenbach T, Edelbrock C: Manual for the Child Behavior Checklist and Revised Child Behavior Profile. Burlington, VT, Thomas M Achenbach, 1983

Asarnow J, Ben-Meirs T, Goldstein M: Family factors in childhood depressive and schizophrenia-spectrum disorders: a preliminary report, in Understanding Major Mental Disorder: The Contribution of Family Interaction Research. Edited by Hahlweg K, Goldstein M. New York, Family Process Press, 1987, pp 123–138

Berg CJ, Rapoport JL, Flament M: The Leyton Obsessional Inventory—Child Version. Psychopharmacol Bull 21:1057–1062, 1985

Conners C: Psychological assessment of children with minimal brain dysfunction. Ann N Y Acad Sci 205:283–302, 1973

Costello EJ, Angold A: Scales to assess child and adolescent depression: checklists, screens, and nets. J Am Acad Child Adolesc Psychiatry 27:726–737, 1988

Cox A, Rutter M: Diagnostic appraisal and interviewing, in Child and Adolescent Psychiatry: Modern Approaches, 2nd Edition. Edited by Rutter M, Hersov L. Oxford, UK, Blackwell Scientific, 1985, pp 233–248

Fann W, Smith R, Davis J, et al: Tardive Dyskinesia: Research and Treatment. Jamaica, NY, Spectrum, 1980

Feist J, Slowiak C, Colligan R: Beyond good intentions: applying scientific methods to the art of milieu therapy. Residential Group Care and Treatment 3:13–32, 1985

Garrison WT, Ecker B, Friedman M, et al: Aggression and counteraggression during child psychiatric hospitalization. J Am Acad Child Adolesc Psychiatry 29:242–250, 1990

Gittelman R: The role of psychological tests for differential diagnosis in child psychiatry. Journal of the American Academy of Child Psychiatry 19:413–438, 1980

Gittelman R: Ratings for anxiety disorders. Psychopharmacol Bull 21:933–948, 1985

Halmi KA, Falk JR, Schwartz E: Binge-eating and vomiting: a survey of a college population. Psychol Med 11:697–706, 1981

Herjanic B, Reich W: Development of a structured psychiatric interview for children: agreement between child and parent on individual symptoms. J Abnorm Child Psychol 10:307–324, 1982

Hodges K, Kline J, Stern L, et al: The development of a child assessment interview for research and clinical use. J Abnorm Child Psychol 10:134–144, 1982

Jones RN, Latkowski ME, Kircher JC, et al: The Child Behavior Checklist: normative information for inpatients. J Am Acad Child Adolesc Psychiatry 27:632–635, 1988

Kolko DJ: Daily ratings on a child psychiatric unit: psychometric evaluation of the Child Behavior Rating Form. J Am Acad Child Adolesc Psychiatry 27:126–132, 1988

Kovacs M: Rating scales to assess depression in school-aged children. Acta Paedopsychiatrica 46:305–315, 1981

Marsden G, McDermott JF, Minor D: Selection of children for residential treatment: a study of evaluation procedures and decision making. Journal of the American Academy of Child Psychiatry 16:427–438, 1977

Matson J, Rotatori A, Helsel W: Development of a rating scale to measure social skills in children: the Matson evaluation of social skills with youngsters. Behaviour Research and Therapy 21:335–340, 1983

McLeer SV, Deblinger E, Atkins MS, et al: Post-traumatic stress disorder in sexually abused children. J Am Acad Child Adolesc Psychiatry 27:650–654,1988

Moos RH: Evaluating Treatment Environments: A Social Ecological Approach. New York, Wiley, 1974

Moos RH, Moos B: Family Environment Scale Manual. Palo Alto, CA, Consulting Psychologists Press, 1981

Orvaschel H, Walsh G: The assessment of adaptive functioning in children: a review of existing measures suitable for epidemiological and clinical services research (DHHS Publ No ADM-84-1343). Washington, DC, U.S. Government Printing Office, 1984

Poznanski E, Cook S, Carroll B: A depression rating scale for children. Pediatrics 64:442–450, 1979

Puig-Antich J, Chambers W: The Schedule for Affective Disorders and Schizophrenia for School-Age Children (Kiddie-SADS). New York, New York State Psychiatric Association, 1978

Raskin J: Assessment of psychopathology by the nurse or psychiatric aide, in The Behavior of Psychiatric Patients: Quantitative Techniques for Evaluation. Edited by Burdock E, Sudilovsky A, Gershon S. New York, Marcel Dekker, 1982, pp 143–176

Ricciuti A, Morton R, Behar D, et al: Medical findings in child psychiatric inpatients. J Am Acad Child Adolesc Psychiatry 26:554–555, 1987

Scharff J: Foundations of Object Relations Family Therapy. Northvale, NJ, Jason Aronson, 1989

Schopler E, Reichler R, Renner B: The Childhood Autism Rating Scale—CARS. New York, Irrington Publications, 1985

Spielberger S: Manual for State-Trait Anxiety Inventory for Children. Palo Alto, CA, Consulting Psychologists Press, 1973

Weller E, Weller R, Fristad M, et al: A potpourri of DST results in prepubertal children. Paper presented at the annual meeting of the American Academy of Child and Adolescent Psychiatry, Chicago, IL, October 1990

Woolston JL, Riddle MA: The role of advanced technology in inpatient child psychiatry: leading edge or useful aid? J Am Acad Child Adolesc Psychiatry 29:905–908, 1990

Chapter 6

Treatment Planning

Treatment planning is naturally derived from the philosophy of treatment and the evaluation process. The treatment plan includes the identification of the major problems within the patient and interpersonal environment, the goals for therapeutic remediation, and specific techniques used to attain stated goals.

There are two principal types of plans formulated during hospitalization. The first, the *long-term treatment plan,* refers to all diagnostic procedures and therapies necessary for as full a remediation of the problems as possible. It includes, but does not limit itself to, the hospitalization portion of the plan. Although the long-term plan is often formulated during hospitalization, some of its components are not fully implemented until after the patient is discharged. The second type is the *focused (hospital) treatment plan* specific to the hospitalization process itself. It outlines the main problem or problems precipitating inpatient care and delineates the specific treatment approaches necessary for discharge and transition to a less restrictive level of care.

Formal treatment planning has been introduced only recently to psychiatry and child psychiatry. During the formative years of inpatient care, therapists used those approaches with which they were comfortable to treat most patient problems. The problems, themselves, were not well delineated, nor were the specific treatment goals and objectives. The impetus for change occurred when Weed (1969) introduced the problem-oriented record to general medicine. During the mid- to late 1970s, psychiatry began the process of treatment planning as we know it today (Cohen 1979; Group for the Advancement of Psychiatry 1973). During the past few years, treatment planning specific to short-term inpatient units has been introduced (Harper 1989; Nurcombe 1989).

Long-Term Treatment Plan

Most patients are hospitalized without previously designed treatment plans. Because one of the main advantages of inpatient care is that it provides the type of data necessary for thorough long-term planning, it is important that the team undertake this process during each patient's hospitalization. Although the initial formulation of the plan is usually undertaken 7 to 10 days following admission, the plan is not finalized until shortly before discharge, because the ongoing collection of data appropriately leads to modification of the originally conceived plan.

The long-term treatment plan, itself, begins with the listing of patient, family, and environmental problems. Each problem is substantiated by objective and subjective data as well as by an assessment integrating the biopsychosocial factors important in precipitating and maintaining the problems. Goals for the therapeutic approach to each problem, as well as stepwise movement toward attainment of the goals (i.e., the measurable objectives), are listed. Finally, specific therapeutic techniques and therapists responsible for each of the patient's problems are recorded.

Case Example

A treatment plan for John, the 10-year-old in the following case example, is presented in Table 6–1.

> John, a 10-year-old, was admitted to our university unit when he refused to return to school following the Christmas holidays because of severe panic-like symptoms when not in the presence of at least one of his parents. Although he had not experienced these symptoms before, he did have an extensive family history of both depression and separation-anxiety disorder. His early development was unremarkable except for undue anxiety and protest associated with separations at the beginning of kindergarten and first grade. Although popular with peers, John had refused in the past to spend the night in the home of friends. His parents said that he whined and pouted and was intermittently oppositional when he did not get his way.
>
> Following the initial presentation of symptoms, the family consulted an outpatient clinician, who subsequently met with the patient, the parents, and the school counselor. Although a reasonable plan for reintroducing John to the classroom was formulated, his extreme anxiety made its implementation impossible. Following 4 days of out-of-control behavior with threats of self-injury, John was referred for inpatient therapy. The initial formulation of his long-term treatment plan was made on the sixth day following admission, when his hospitalization plan was also formulated. The plan was not finalized, however, until shortly before discharge, 3 weeks after admission.

Table 6–1. Long-term treatment plan for John, a 10-year-old (see case example)

PROBLEM I: Panic-like behavior at times of separation

Data: Anxiety, crying, out-of-control behavior, threats of self-injury; family history of depression and separation anxiety; developmental history of wariness at times of separation; paternal therapeutic response to desipramine 3 years prior to the patient's development of symptoms.

CBCL results include schizoid-anxious scale, 5 (greater than 98th percentile); somatic complaints scale, 3.5 (just under 98th percentile).

Patient strengths include intelligence and academic achievement, reasonably good peer relationships, a desire for symptom relief, and family support.

Assessment: The patient has a biological proclivity toward separation anxiety and exhibits symptoms consistent with separation-anxiety disorder. Somatization symptoms are prominent.

Goal: The incapacitating nature of the symptoms will be reduced so that John will be able to return to school and to normal functioning.

Objectives

1. A decrease of symptoms sufficient for the patient to attend school on the inpatient unit.
2. Generalization of gains to the posthospitalization treatment setting as measured by John's behavior during passes home and following discharge.
3. For John to return to school following discharge and remain in school without significant exacerbation of his separation anxiety.

Plan

1. Alliance-building individual psychotherapy, designed to foster the development of trust, to formulate a dynamic understanding of the patient's psychopathology, and to give the patient a forum to discuss his subjective feelings about his situation. (*Duration:* during hospitalization.)
2. **Pharmacotherapy:** Start desipramine after an electrocardiogram has been obtained and reported as normal. Increase the dose by increments of 25 mg until the patient is taking 75 mg per day; at that point, order a desipramine blood level and modify dosage accordingly; use 0.25 mg of alprazolam as needed to manage untoward anxiety symptoms; monitor for side effects.
3. **Milieu therapy:** Staff will establish an alliance to help increase patient sense of security and to maintain safety by managing out-of-control behaviors. John

Table 6–1. Long-term treatment plan for John, a 10-year-old (see case example) (continued)

will attend the unit school on the second day following admission. A child care worker will accompany John to the unit classroom and will remain with him throughout the first week.

PROBLEM II: Nonassertive, passive behaviors

Data: John presents with fearful, overcontrolled behaviors and very little use of appropriate assertiveness. His parents are overly solicitous of his wishes as they inadvertently reinforce John's passivity. John often asks his parents to manage situations that he could easily handle. CBCL social withdrawal scale on teacher report, 4 (90th percentile); internalizing scale, 31 (greater than 98th percentile).

Assessment: John is developing personality traits indicative of passivity. His parents are reinforcing these traits. His behaviors serve to exercise control over his parents and to avoid appropriate psychological separation.

Goal: The patient will develop more assertive ways of achieving individual goals and desires. John will become more appropriately autonomous and will psychologically separate from his parents. John's parents will stop reinforcing the development of his passive personality traits.

Objectives (during hospitalization)

1. The patient will give up whining, complaining behaviors when making requests of staff members.
2. The patient will be able to negotiate directly with his therapist for home passes, without asking for parent intervention.
3. John's parents will develop rules for expected behavior within their home.

Plan

1. **Individual therapy:** John will meet with the individual therapist two times per week for initial alliance building and then to explore his psychological development, including perception of self, internal object structures, and his use of defense mechanisms. The relationship between these facets and his symptoms and behaviors will be formulated. Interpretations and treatment strategies will be developed accordingly.[a] (*Duration:* at least 12 months.)
2. **Behavior therapy:** The activities therapist will meet with the patient two times per week and employ cognitive-behavioral therapy and assertiveness training designed to help John learn to use more direct, assertive behaviors to achieve his goals. (*Duration:* during hospitalization.)
3. **Group therapy:** John will attend daily activity-interview group sessions designed to teach him how to delay gratification and increase frustration toler-

Table 6–1. Long-term treatment plan for John, a 10-year-old (see case example) (continued)

ance, as well as assertiveness training techniques. (*Duration:* during hospitalization.)

4. **Milieu techniques:** Unit child care workers and nursing staff members will reward increased assertiveness taught in individual and group therapy while managing issues of daily living.

5. **Parent training:** Parents will attend parent training sessions ($1\frac{1}{2}$ hours per week) designed to help them learn to establish rules and set limits within the home, to establish consequences for infractions of the rules, and to apply the stated consequences. (*Duration:* 8 weeks.)

6. John's parents will work on the unit with child care workers 3 hours per week learning skills to promote assertive behavior.[b]

PROBLEM III: Family dysfunction

Data: John's parents spend little time exclusively with each other. John's father has an explosive temper when frustrated and a history of depression successfully treated with desipramine. John's two siblings are also described by parents as intrusive and difficult to discipline.

Assessment: There are problems with intimacy between the parents. One of the patient's roles in the family is to come between his parents to camouflage the problems with their intimacy.

Goal

1. Parents will be able to understand their contributions to the patient's problems and their own issues regarding interpersonal intimacy.

2. John's father will be able to present with more appropriately assertive behavior and fewer temper outbursts.

Objectives

1. The parents will spend at least one night per week together without the children.

2. John's father will be able to go for at least 1 week without an angry temper tantrum.

Plan

1. **Family therapy:** Family will meet once per week for a limited number of sessions in structural family therapy designed to help remove the children from the parental hierarchy.

Table 6–1. Long-term treatment plan for John, a 10-year-old (see case example) (continued)

2. **Couples therapy:** Parents will meet for 1 hour per week in couples therapy designed to examine their conflicts about intimacy and to begin to deal with their sexual difficulties. (*Duration:* at least 6 months—to begin after family sessions have begun.)

3. **Individual therapy evaluation** (for the father): This is designed to examine the issues related to the father's passivity and to his explosive temper. (*Duration:* not predetermined.)

PROBLEM IV. School

Data: John presents with perfectionistic tendencies in the classroom. His academic achievement is above average. When a staff member visited John's regular classroom, the teacher was observed to be stern and demanding toward students. John also expressed a fear of the teacher.

Assessment: The patient's anxiety about school is definitely increased by both his own perfectionism and his fear of the teacher. There is a poor patient-teacher fit.

Goal: The school principal and teacher will understand how the patient's anxieties are increased by these classroom issues.

Objectives

1. The team will understand the teacher's perspective on the problems.
2. The school counselor and the teacher will agree to work with the treatment team to discuss how to form an alliance with the patient.
3. The teacher will agree to examine ways in which she can positively reinforce and reward John in the classroom for appropriate behavior.

Plan

1. The treatment team will meet with the principal, school counselor, and teacher to discuss their views regarding the origins of John's problems as well as what needs to be done for John to return to school.
2. The teacher will meet with the treatment team to discuss problems between John and her and objectives for improving their relationship (during week 2 of hospitalization).
3. The school counselor and teacher will meet with the parents to discuss ongoing ways of working together (prior to and following discharge).

Note: CBCL = Child Behavior Checklist (Achenbach and Edelbrock 1983).
[a]See case of Matt in Chapter 7.
[b]See Chapter 11.

Hospitalization Treatment Plan

The purpose of the hospitalization treatment plan is to move the patient as efficiently as possible to a less restrictive treatment setting that will foster psychological growth (Nurcombe 1989). The team meets during the first week following admission to formulate this plan. Following the evaluation, a diagnostic formulation summarizing the biological, intrapsychic, interpersonal, and environmental factors precipitating and maintaining the problematic behaviors is outlined as described in the long-term plan above (see Table 6–1). Pivotal problems are then extracted. Simply stated, these are the symptoms that must change for movement to a less restrictive level of care. Next, goals, primarily related to patient stabilization, are devised. Then, treatment approaches necessary to attain the goals are chosen. A target date is set for accomplishment of the objectives, and a means of evaluating the success of the plan is chosen. A discharge plan, which includes the posthospitalization therapy approach and level of care, as well as the necessary liaison work, follows. The entire plan is discussed with the patient and family. It is implemented, monitored, and revised as necessary. Finally, the patient is discharged (Nurcombe 1989).

Most recently, Harper (1989) has offered an alternative approach to Nurcombe's goal-directed planning. Harper's method, termed *focal inpatient treatment planning,* differs by emphasizing a single problem and formulating it in operational language, by inviting a comprehensive discussion of pathogenesis, by including the input of the environment and patient strengths, and by using language that is jargon-free.

In our experience, a combination of these two approaches has provided the best results. A thorough diagnostic formulation, the identification of a single, pivotal problem, and clearly stated goals and therapeutic approaches, as well as a statement of patient, family, and environmental strengths, are the most useful components for efficient planning.

In John's case (see case example above), the evaluation data extracted from the long-term plan described in Table 6–1 led to the development of a focused hospitalization treatment plan, as shown in Table 6–2.

This system of problem-oriented planning requires a highly organized team approach. By focusing team members on specific problems, therapeutic approaches, and target dates, this type of planning helps to minimize the possibility of inefficient delivery of inpatient services. On the other hand, by formulating both focused and long-term plans during hospitalization, the team has the necessary ingredients at hand for more in-depth work if environmental and patient factors conspire to make posthospitalization progress unlikely. Furthermore, by extracting the pivotal problems and therapeutic approaches in the focused plan from the long-term treatment plan, the former fits neatly into the latter, contributing to a smooth transition from the hospital. The organization implicit in these approaches facilitates the handling of third-party payer and research issues.

John was discharged 19 days following admission. Although anxious on the first day of his return to school, he was able to attend classes and, by the third day, was reasonably reintegrated into school. John, his parents, and

Table 6–2. Focused hospitalization treatment plan for John, a 10-year-old (see case example)

1. **Pivotal problem:** Panic-like symptoms when separated from his parents, leading to disabling anxiety and threats of self-injury.
2. **Diagnostic formulation:** John suffers with a biological proclivity toward major affective disorder and separation-anxiety disorder that acts as a strong predisposing factor for his symptoms. His parents' marital difficulties, his father's characterological problems, and the parents' inability to reasonably limit his behaviors have strongly served to maintain his difficulties. His postvacation anxiety about school and his fear of the teacher's stern approach have served as major precipitants. Finally, John's family's response to his separation-anxiety symptoms has reinforced and perpetuated the presenting behaviors.
3. **Strengths:** Patient's desire for symptom relief, his intelligence, and his peer relationships.
4. **Stabilization goals:** To sufficiently manage the underlying biological contributants to the symptoms; to reduce the parents' overindulgent and solicitous attitude, which assists in maintaining the problem; and to encourage the teacher to adopt a different approach with the patient.
5. **Specific objectives:** John will be able to return to school without a recurrence of incapacitating symptoms, and his parents and staff at school will be able to reinforce healthy behavior.
6. **Therapy approaches (interventions):** Stabilization on desipramine and use of alprazolam as necessary; stabilization of patient within the milieu; alliance-building psychotherapy; family therapy; parent training sessions; parent involvement within the milieu therapy program; and coordination planning with school personnel. These approaches are all aimed at the attunement of fit between patient and interpersonal environment. [Names of unit personnel who are responsible for therapies should be specified in plan.]
7. **Target date:** Patient should be ready for discharge to home 3 weeks following admission.
8. **Discharge plan:** Return to home; outpatient individual therapy and desipramine for John; family therapy; referral of father for individual therapy [specify name(s) of therapist(s)]; attendance in regular classroom. Regular diet and no restriction on activity [these items required by accreditation agencies].

his father continued in outpatient psychotherapy for 14 months following discharge. His desipramine was discontinued after 7 months. Two years following discharge, the patient and his family were doing well.

Discharge Plan

One of the major purposes of focused treatment planning is to prepare the treatment team for patient discharge. The team must talk about and formulate an actual plan detailing the termination process and posthospitalization therapies. This is accomplished as soon as the posthospitalization level of care necessary for continued growth is determined.

If the plan is for the patient and family to continue to work with the hospital team following discharge, planning for the transition from the hospital is fairly simple. In these situations, the clinician and family discuss and determine a discharge date and follow-up plan that is subsequently implemented. The termination process includes a discussion of posthospitalization treatment goals, contingency plans if problems recur, therapeutic passes to practice newly learned behaviors, management of separation and termination issues within the milieu, and the actual discharge.

If the postdischarge plan involves referral of the patient and family, communication must be timely and precise. The hospital clinician reviews with the future therapist the major issues and understandings gained about the patient, family, and environment during hospitalization. The ability of the patient and family to establish therapeutic alliances and to work productively, as well as the short-term and long-term treatment goals, are discussed in detail. Evaluations, treatment plans, and treatment summaries are sent to the future therapist as soon as possible.

If discharge to home is not feasible, then other-than-home discharge placements are chosen as early as possible during the hospitalization process. The information mentioned above is sent to the facility (e.g., state hospital, residential facility) in a timely manner. The family and patient are encouraged to visit the facility during the patient's hospitalization, when possible. Treatment team members of the future treating facility are encouraged to attend hospital staffings and to observe the patient within the unit milieu. The hospital clinician reviews the patient's long-term treatment goals and needs with the future facility to ensure treatment continuity. When the patient is in state custody and parents are not available, members of the treatment team physically accompany the patient from the hospital unit to the next placement, when possible. (The termination process in such instances will be discussed in Chapter 12.)

The lack of an appropriate discharge placement necessary for continued patient growth confounds the entire discharge process, as discussed in

Chapter 2 (see section on length of stay). This lack of appropriate placement reflects the contemporary breakdown in family, social, and community resources and presents a very difficult problem for public patients with special needs. It is also a problem, however, for those private patients with limited third-party payer coverage who cannot afford posthospitalization treatment, or whose benefits expire during the course of hospitalization. In these cases, the clinician and the hospital have a responsibility to continue inpatient treatment until a posthospitalization treatment approach with a reasonable potential for fostering developmental growth can be found or until a transfer of the patient to a public facility can be obtained.

It is incumbent on the clinician and the hospital prior to admission to estimate the level of the patient's needs in conjunction with the family's economic resources. When the decision is made to hospitalize, the clinician and hospital commit themselves to providing the services necessary for the reestablishment of positive developmental growth. Abruptly discharging patients who can no longer afford inpatient care prior to the attainment of stated goals is unethical.

Staffings

The treatment team meets together at least once, but preferably twice, per week to discuss patient progress, treatment, and staff concerns. Treatment plans are devised and revised during the staffing sessions. Staffings are essential in maintaining the type of communication and contact necessary for the milieu to function therapeutically. (See Chapter 15 for a discussion of treatment team composition.)

The team leader chairs the meetings. Each patient's progress in the various therapies is discussed. The teacher reports on academic and behavioral performance in the unit school program. Information is shared and movement toward treatment goals is assessed. Finally, treatment approaches are altered as necessary.

All treatment team members attend at least one staffing per week. Agency workers sometimes attend these meetings, as do posthospitalization therapists, to become familiar with the treatment plan and to coordinate the patient's transition from the hospital. Although mandated in some settings, inclusion of the patient or family in the staffing process has not, in our experience, been found profitable because it frequently impedes discussion. Although the involvement of the patient and family in the organization and implementation of the plan is vital, it has been our experience that this can be most readily facilitated during individual and family therapy sessions.

In addition to the above-stated purpose of staffings (i.e., to foster communication among team members), it is also important that the team leader use these meetings to synthesize and integrate the presented data in such a way that the dynamic issues make sense to team members. Staffings are most productive when they impart an understanding of what is going on and how the chosen therapy approaches are designed to address the problems.

Progress Notes

Progress notes also facilitate communication. They should be designed to continually update the chart on how the patient is moving toward the stated treatment goals. The SOAP (subjective data, objective data, assessment, plan) or DAP (data, assessment, plan) format is used in child psychiatry charts for the same reasons it is used on medical and surgical services (see Table 6–3). This format encourages specificity and keeps the treatment goals and objectives in focus. Overly detailed notes describing the process of individual or family sessions are unnecessary unless the information provided clarifies progress toward stated goals.

Each therapist should write a note following each therapy session. Furthermore, the team leader should write daily notes coordinating the presented data, substantiating the diagnostic formulation, assessing movement toward the goals, describing changes in therapeutic approaches, and detailing pharmacotherapy side effects. Although this might seem excessive, the chart must note that the patient is therapeutically seen each day and must describe how the approaches used are moving the patient toward treatment goals.

Progress notes are especially important when reviewing patient evaluation and treatment following discharge. This process is often necessary for both research and medicolegal reasons. The above-mentioned guidelines greatly facilitate the substantiation of quality care when the provision of services is questioned following hospitalization.

Confounding Issues

A major issue impeding adequate treatment planning is the difficulty implicit in reducing extensive patient, family, and environmental data into the above-described framework. Effectively summarizing all of the pertinent clinical information and organizing it so that it is both useful and efficiently stated can be a frustrating and time-consuming task. However, if done well, a comprehensive and cohesive treatment plan can be invaluable for a good treatment outcome.

The most common confounding issue regarding treatment planning, however, is when the process is not taken seriously. Because of accreditation purposes or hospital policies, treatment teams sometimes undertake the process in pro forma fashion. When this happens, team members go through the motions necessary for planning but do not seriously use the process in clinically rewarding ways, and various interventions take on a formula-like approach.

Finally, most treatment teams do not develop both long-term and more focused hospitalization treatment plans. Because hospitalization is often seen as solely short term, teams overlook the potential benefits that accrue from long-term planning. By sidestepping this process, the team misses a chance to use generated inpatient data to effectively coordinate long-term goals and treatment approaches for the patient and family.

Table 6–3. Progress notes: an example of the SOAP and DAP formats

Problem 1: Depression manifested by suicidal ideation, sleep and appetite disturbance, crying spells

SOAP[a]

Date Problem # 1
Time

S: "I don't feel too good today."

O: Patient appears sad. Talks about separation from family. Has been sleeping poorly at night, only 2 hours/night. No evidence of suicidal ideation. Most recent desipramine level = 40.

A: Depression persists. No change from last visit.

P: Continue psychotherapy. Talk to social worker about family involvement. Increase desipramine to 25 mg tid. Repeat level in 2 weeks.

DAP[b]

Date Problem # 1
Time 9:00 A.M.

D: Patient says he doesn't feel well today. Appeared sad. Talks about separation from family. Has been sleeping poorly at night, only 2 hours/night. No evidence of suicidal ideation. Most recent desipramine level = 40.

A: Depression persists. No change from last visit.

P: Continue psychotherapy. Talk to social worker about family involvement. Increase desipramine to 25 mg tid. Repeat level in 2 weeks.

[a]Subjective data, objective data, assessment, plan.
[b]Data, assessment, plan.

References

Achenbach T, Edelbrock C: Manual for the Child Behavior Checklist and Revised Child Behavior Profile. Burlington, VT, Thomas M Achenbach, 1983

Cohen RL: Case formulation and treatment planning, in Basic Handbook of Child Psychiatry, Vol 1. Edited by Call JD, Noshpitz JD, Cohen RL, et al (JD Noshpitz, Editor-in-Chief). New York, Basic Books, 1979, pp 485–504

Group for the Advancement of Psychiatry: From Diagnosis to Treatment, Vol 8, Report No 87. New York, Group for the Advancement of Psychiatry, 1973

Harper G: Focal inpatient treatment planning. J Am Acad Child Adolesc Psychiatry 28:31–37, 1989

Nurcombe B: Goal-directed treatment planning and the principles of brief hospitalization. J Am Acad Child Adolesc Psychiatry 28:26–30, 1989

Weed L: Medical Records, Medical Evaluation and Patient Care. Cleveland, OH, Case Western Reserve University Press, 1969

Chapter 7

Individual Psychotherapy

Although once considered the cornerstone of inpatient treatment, the current use of individual psychotherapy during hospitalization is being rigorously questioned. Our belief is that when indicated and well implemented, it can substantially contribute to patient progress. There are various purposes for the general use of individual psychotherapy, including symptom reduction, promotion of normal development, fostering of autonomy and self-reliance, and the generalization of behavioral gains (Rutter 1985). In addition, purposes specific to inpatient work include providing information for the formation and revision of the long-term treatment plan as well as elucidating the unconscious motivations for the patient's problematic behaviors.

Although basically similar, inpatient individual psychotherapy differs from outpatient therapy in several ways. As Greenwood (1955) has pointed out, inpatient therapy occurs within a social atmosphere in which patients talk among themselves about the therapy process and their therapists. Patients become familiar with personal characteristics of therapists through direct observation and by listening to others in a way that rarely happens during outpatient treatment. They soon discover that their therapists know about their milieu behavior. Their inability to hide this behavior has significant transference implications, as the individual therapist may be seen as all knowing, omnipotent, punitive, or gratifying. Also, the therapist's involvement in the patient's day-to-day unit life can contribute to both increased dependence and oppositionalism.

Furthermore, inpatient therapists share themes from the patient's individual psychotherapy with team members to clarify the self-related issues contributing to the mis-fit between patient and environment. This knowledge is vital for the treatment planning process. Before this is done, however, confidentiality is discussed with the patient. The reasons for sharing personal data with team members are offered, and the child is reassured that specific details elaborated during psychotherapy about past life events do not have to be spelled out for team members. For example, although it is important to share information about past sexual abuse and subsequent feelings and reactions, the description of what specifically happened during the sexual abuse is confidential. The problems that this policy might potentially cause regarding the development of trust can usually be managed supportively.

In outpatient work, the therapist is the center of the treatment plan, whereas during hospitalization he or she is only one member of a larger clinical team. This sharing of responsibility sometimes creates problems for those clinicians who are more accustomed to outpatient work. All team members must be alert for the possibility of splitting by the patient, which is a frequent consequence when an individual therapist is working with multiple caregivers.

One of the main advantages of inpatient psychotherapy is its intensity. Individual sessions three to five times per week, in concert with other forms of therapy, and day-to-day treatment within the milieu can be very effective in hastening the reparative process. In some cases, psychological problems requiring extensive outpatient treatment respond well to intensive short- or medium-term hospital psychotherapy.

There are many styles and types of psychotherapy. Two important categories, supportive and dynamic, are frequently used during hospitalization, the former to provide support and build alliances while other therapeutic interventions are employed.

Supportive Psychotherapy

During supportive psychotherapy the therapist directly helps the patient relate to unit staff, handle the limits imposed within the milieu, and adapt to changes within the unit routine, including the eventual termination process. The therapist seeks to clarify the environmental issues causing problems for the patient and helps in the development of more adaptive ways of managing these problems. Reassurance and the provision of nurturance are essential, as well as very clear limit setting with consequences based on the patient's developmental level and psychological functioning. This approach is especially useful in combination with biological, group, or behavioral therapies.

It is important to keep in mind, however, that supportive therapy does not preclude the use of strategies and techniques often reserved for dynamic psychotherapy. During the course of hospitalization, psychological conflicts often surface, even in patients with developmental disabilities, psychosis, mental retardation, or other seriously limiting conditions. Dynamic issues should be addressed in developmentally appropriate ways during these times, using play therapy with younger children and play and verbal approaches with older children.

Dynamic Psychotherapy

Traditional dynamic psychotherapy is also frequently used during hospitalization. It is more often indicated for attainment of the goals that are defined in the long-term treatment plan than of those in the focused inpatient treatment plan. However, the implementation of individual psychotherapy, even during a relatively brief hospitalization, may offer considerable benefit to some patients.

Dynamic psychotherapy is designed to correct the child's problematic sense of self when it is a major contributant to the patient-environment mis-fit. This deficit in the sense of self, in the absence of accompanying organic symptomatology, is most often a product of unresolved early trauma and interpersonal and psychological conflict. It is manifested in patients with borderline personality traits and other pathological characteristics; cases of posttraumatic stress disorders secondary to abuse; many cases of conduct disorder, affective disorder, and anxiety disorder; and patients with oppositional disorder (Terr 1991). It is also manifested in acting-out children from psychologically disturbed, rigid families (Terr 1991). We think that, when indicated, the therapy described in this section, in concert with other therapies, can significantly enhance the long-term outcome of the patient. In our experience, this approach is appropriate for about one-third of the patients in both our university unit and the state hospital unit.

Dynamic psychotherapy usually involves the gradual verbalization of the elements related to the patient's psychological trauma and conflicts in the past, which contribute to current behavior and mood states. The loss of important objects, recurring abuse, and unresolved trauma secondary to inadequate, ungratifying attachments and multiple separation experiences frequently hamper healthy growth and contribute to the subsequent development of character pathology (van der Kolk 1989). Individual psychotherapy provides the opportunity for the patient to examine how these past traumas are reenacted interpersonally, what underlying feelings contribute to this reenactment, how to express those feelings differently and thus interrupt the pathological repetition, and how to direct internal energies in a positive fashion. This approach borrows elements from both open-ended and time-limited therapy with children. Although the process is allowed to develop, the therapist plays an active role by gently but consistently pointing out how the patient's verbalizations and behaviors relate to the underlying problems.

Phases of Dynamic Psychotherapy

There are various discrete phases of individual dynamic psychotherapy that are relevant to the hospitalization process (Table 7–1):

Alliance building. The first phase includes alliance building (i.e., the building of trust). The therapist provides a secure working environment and allows the patient to set the agenda during the first several sessions. This corresponds with the patient's "honeymoon" phase. After five or six sessions, however, the therapist begins to make connections between the presented material and the underlying problems. This usually leads to objections and subsequent resistance on the patient's part, which are interpreted and gently confronted by reminding the patient how these resistances and problematic behaviors have continually led to difficulties in the past.

Confrontation of the problem. Confrontation of the problem may provoke more symptomatology within the milieu and, sometimes, in the therapy sessions as well. This second phase often consists of a reenactment of the original trauma within the transference. Negative transference must be addressed by the therapist during this period, neither allowing it to stalemate the treatment nor providing an arena for the patient to continually act out the original problems. Patients often swing between anger and sadness, although it is usually difficult for these patients to allow themselves to experience depression for a significant period of time. The therapist empathizes with the patient's dilemma and suggests that these feelings are also a product of early developmental issues and events. The therapist uses the patient's play and verbalizations to understand the important areas of conflict and enlists the patient's help in connecting negative affect with important events and situations. The patient's real wishes (and real self) are gleaned. Cognitive-behavioral interventions (Sloves and Peterlin 1986) are often used at this time to help minimize negative transference (see Chapter 9). The patient is taught coping strategies that enhance autonomous ego functions (e.g., the ability to delay gratification, anticipation, reflection, problem solving).

Working through. Working through has been identified as a critical therapeutic phase (Kennedy 1982). During this time the patient's conflict becomes more internalized and is less likely to be acted out within the milieu.

Table 7–1. Phases of individual dynamic psychotherapy

1. Alliance building	3. Working through
2. Confrontation of the problem	4. Internalization

Patients experience more reasonable affect and transference manifestations as the therapist's autonomy and separateness become increasingly accepted. As this phase takes hold, patients begin to view their own behaviors and negative affective states as products of internal, unresolved issues as opposed to being someone else's fault. This decreasing externalization of affect and behavior corresponds with an increasing trust in the therapist and the therapy process.

Internalization. During the final phase, internalization (Kennedy 1982), there is an application of what has been learned in therapy to new, potentially stressful situations. The patient becomes less vulnerable to everyday conflicts that previously had precipitated behaviors and mood states, such as those precipitating hospitalization. During this phase, patients learn to recognize current events that usually upset them and to develop more adaptive strategies for handling these situations.

In order to attain the therapy goals, the patient and therapist meet together in individual therapy three to five times per week during hospitalization. Just as in the milieu, the individual therapist must use a balance between limit setting and the provision of nurturance. Knowing when to confront, when to use empathy, when to remain silent, and when to delve into the patient's past is essential for a positive outcome. Strategies and techniques used to build therapeutic relationships and to assist in affective repair are the cornerstones of this work. We have attempted to highlight them in this chapter, but they can only be fully learned through supervision with experienced inpatient psychotherapists.

Termination

Discharge from the hospital may occur at various points during the individual therapy process. Although the discharge date depends on a number of issues, hopefully the patient's progress in individual therapy will be considered. For those patients who will continue to work in posthospitalization individual therapy with their hospital therapist, discharge from the standpoint of psychotherapy is appropriate after a reasonable alliance has been formed and presenting symptoms have been successfully contained. For those patients who will have a different posthospitalization therapist, discharge ideally should be delayed until the patient has begun the rudimentary process of internalization accompanied by a diminution of symptoms.

Regardless of when discharge occurs during the therapy process, there is a termination process that must be considered. Patients require time to work through the separation and loss implicit in discharge. Although leaving the security of the hospital is difficult in and of itself, it also consciously and unconsciously reminds the patient of previous psychological separations and losses that have not been adequately resolved.

Frequently, when the discharge date is set, patients who earlier during treatment had begun to control their problematic behavior seem to lose those controls. There is a recycling process in which the recurrence of symptomatic behavior requires the type of limit setting used during the initial part of hospitalization. It is as though patients need reassurances that their previously disruptive behavior will be adequately managed by caregivers outside of the hospital. This interpretation frequently serves to limit this recycling and to help the patient focus on separation and termination issues.

Case Example

Matt, 9 years of age, was admitted to our university unit with periods of extreme oppositionalism and an extensive history of tantrum-like behavior when his wishes were not fulfilled. Matt had no friends because of his frequent physical fights. He continually demanded attention and was unable to spend time alone. He had run away from home and from foster placements on eight occasions, was very overactive, and, prior to hospitalization, had seriously attempted suicide. He exhibited no biological signs or symptoms indicative of depression, denied hallucinations and frank delusions, presented with no pressured speech or other symptoms indicative of mania (except possibly for intermittent overactivity), and was in the above-average range of intelligence. He did have a cleft palate, about which he frequently complained.

Matt's mother had died shortly after his birth. He was reared by a sadistic father who frequently abused and neglected him until he was 4 years old, at which time he went to live with his paternal grandmother. His father remarried and lived with his new family only a short distance from the patient and his grandmother. Matt envied his new siblings who were definitely favored by the father. When he became increasingly aggressive in his grandmother's home, he went to live with his father and stepmother. Because of subsequent physical abuse and possible sexual abuse, the state assumed custody and placed Matt in a foster home, where he seriously acted out. After placement in several residential facilities where he was treated with antipsychotics and lithium carbonate, his aggressive acting out increased and he exhibited multiple, discrete psychotic episodes. His state social worker then moved him to a very secure therapeutic foster home with the hopes that the environmental stability and structure would lead to a reduction of symptoms. Although there was some improvement, the patient's continuing physical aggression and unpredictable mood states jeopardized the placement. Outpatient therapy, pharmacotherapy, and parent training had not stabilized the situation sufficiently so that Matt could remain within the therapeutic foster home. Matt's social worker referred him for hospitalization for a thorough evaluation, treatment planning, and individual and family therapy, hoping for adequate change so that Matt would be able to return to the foster family.

Matt was diagnosed as having posttraumatic stress disorder and attention-deficit hyperactivity disorder combined with conduct disorder, as well as borderline personality traits. The data strongly supported the assessment that Matt's aggressive behavior was a reaction to the profound psychological rejection and lack of supportive and nurturing parenting to which he had been subjected during his formative years. He had also inherited a very difficult temperament, which contributed to the symptom pattern. His multiple placements within abusive and insensitive environments further compounded his problems.

Matt's strengths included his intelligence, his desire for satisfying relationships, and his new foster family. His foster mother, whose own father had had chronic bipolar illness, was very committed to providing an appropriately structured, long-term living environment for the patient. Although her rescue fantasies did complicate matters, her wish to help provided the stability necessary for the type of long-term psychotherapy outlined in the treatment plan.

Alliance building. During the first week of hospitalization, Matt's previously noted symptoms did not emerge. He followed the rules, was very passive with peers, and generally strove to earn all of his level system points. He eagerly attended individual therapy daily. Although readily engaged within the play process, he avoided discussion of either his feelings or his past, the same way he avoided interpersonal conflict within the milieu.

At the end of the first week, the patient's defenses began to weaken. During quiet time on the fifth day following admission, Matt asked if he could watch television, an activity not allowed at that time. When denied, he responded with verbal abuse and, subsequently, physical abuse, requiring time out and physical restraint. During the following therapy session, when asked about the disturbance, Matt responded with oppositionalism and reticence. Matt's therapist made the connection between his unfulfilled wishes and subsequent behavior. When Matt then became aggressive within the session, the therapist explained that limits would be set and that his behavior would not lead to rejection. The therapist's statement of the problem and subsequent reassurance that the symptoms and behaviors would not sabotage the developing relationship brought the first phase of psychotherapy to an end. Matt's behavior on the unit continued to be intermittently disruptive.

Confrontation of the problem. The second phase of psychotherapy—confrontation of the problem—lasted 5 to 6 weeks. During this period, Matt insisted on playing the role of a puppy while the therapist played the role of the puppy's mother. Within this metaphor, he strove to obtain nurturance and avoid conflict. It was another attempt on his part to create the type of symbiotic union he felt was necessary for nurturance (Mahler et al. 1975). When this was directly interpreted and thus interrupted, he became very upset. It was as though he was again reliving the deprivation he experienced early in life.

After providing structure and support, the therapist helped Matt see that the interruption of his wishes for direct gratification was not a rebuff and that there were ways for Matt to have his needs met other than via an idealized fantasy reunion with mother (while rejecting available caregivers). Matt's acting out of these wishes in therapy was likened to other unit and prehospitalization behaviors and was verbally interpreted as the patient's misguided attempt to have his needs met. This phase came to an end as the patient became more able to hear interpretations without subsequent rage and resistance.

Working through. Slowly Matt's limit testing and aggressive unit behaviors diminished. He stopped his insistent begging for attention. In therapy, the play revolved around a mythical family with a very attractive, intelligent, and popular younger son. This led to a discussion about his own dysmorphic features and the disorganizing, negative affect associated with them. A period of depression followed during which time the therapist and patient talked about more productive ways of dealing with needs (e.g., asking for time with his foster parents, working with his primary child care worker on a special school project).

Matt was discharged during this working-through phase, 10 weeks following admission. After the discharge date was announced, almost 3 weeks prior to discharge, the patient immediately regressed within the milieu and became resistant in therapy. He insisted that he was pleased with his approaching discharge and that he would not miss anyone whom he had met at the hospital. His defenses against the fear of abandonment and sadness were interpreted, and he was reassured that he and the therapist would continue to work together, initially on a three-times-per-week basis, following hospitalization. The patient responded fairly well to this approach and was discharged as planned.

Although some of Matt's previously described behaviors reappeared following discharge, their frequency and intensity were diminished sufficiently so that with reasonable structure, he was maintained within his foster home. In the fall he attended a new school. At first, he treated his peers in a bossy fashion and was subsequently rejected by them. With continued therapy, however, he came to recognize that his behavior in school was yet another example of his reaction to anxiety over peer acceptance. When he was subsequently able to modify his reactions, his peer relations improved.

Internalization. In therapy, Matt alternated between playing the role of the perfect son within the mythical family and discussing his reasons for low self-esteem. He slowly came to understand the patterns of his feelings and subsequent behaviors. His frenetic behavior had served as both an attempt to gain acceptance and an angry reaction to the rejection that he perceived. Matt was well into this fourth therapy phase when he was consistently able to alter his previous pattern of acting out. He continued in therapy for 2 years following discharge.

Although not previously stated, the coordination of therapies by Matt's individual therapist during the hospitalization process was very important for his recovery. Parent training and family therapy were vital for his foster parents to understand their own motivations and to be able to place reasonable limits on Matt's behavior. School liaison work was necessary for Matt's transition back to school. Assertiveness training taught Matt how to understand and ask for what he needed and wanted. Group therapy provided important feedback without psychologically flooding the patient. The milieu helped him gain self-control by providing a secure holding environment, despite his attempts to reenact the original traumas by trying to provoke caregivers. Without this coordinated approach, individual therapy would not have been successful.

Confounding Issues

Many clinicians and researchers have reasoned that because the goal of contemporary hospitalization is behavioral management and stabilization, the need to "understand the unconscious" during hospitalization is unnecessary (Hersov and Bentovim 1985). We believe, however, that the clinician and treatment team miss a valuable opportunity to understand key internal issues in some patients if individual dynamic psychotherapy is not pursued. Understanding these issues can be vital to the success of long-term treatment planning, a major goal for all hospitalizations.

Individual therapy is frequently overlooked on both public and private school-age units where there are either too many patients or not enough skilled therapists. These deficiencies will affect the provision of supportive psychotherapy as well as dynamically oriented approaches, setting the stage for more acting out by patients. The acting-out behaviors demand staff attention in the management of crises, further reducing the amount of time available for psychotherapy.

On the other hand, dynamic psychotherapy may sometimes be over-applied to all conditions and situations. Clinicians with a bias toward dynamic psychotherapy sometimes fail during the evaluation process to fully comprehend the influence of particular biological vulnerabilities and social factors seriously contributing to the pathology in some patients. Exclusively applying this technique to the treatment of, for example, aggressive conduct disorders often leads to unsatisfying results.

References

Greenwood ED: The role of residential treatment for children: the role of psychotherapy in residential treatment. Am J Orthopsychiatry 25:692–698, 1955

Hersov L, Bentovim A: In-patient and day-hospital units, in Child and Adolescent Psychiatry: Modern Approaches, 2nd Edition. Edited by Rutter M, Hersov L. Oxford, UK, Blackwell Scientific, 1985, pp 766–779

Kennedy PA: Phases of milieu therapy, in Psychiatric Hospitalization of Children. Edited by Schulman JL, Irwin M. Springfield, IL, Charles C Thomas, 1982, pp 119–128

Mahler MS, Pine F, Bergman A: The Psychological Birth of the Human Infant: Symbiosis and Individuation. New York, Basic Books, 1975

Rutter M: Psychological therapies in child psychiatry: issues and progress, in Child and Adolescent Psychiatry, 2nd Edition. Edited by Rutter M, Hersov L. Oxford, UK, Blackwell Scientific, 1985, pp 927–940

Sloves R, Peterlin KB: The process of time-limited psychotherapy with latency-aged children. J Am Acad Child Adolesc Psychiatry 25:847–851, 1986

Terr L: Childhood traumas: an outline and overview. Am J Psychiatry 148:10–20, 1991

van der Kolk BA: The compulsion to repeat the trauma: re-enactment, revictimization, and masochism. Psychiatr Clin North Am 12:389–411, 1989

Chapter 8

Psychopharmacotherapy

The development of pediatric psychopharmacology occurred following the introduction of amphetamines for disturbed children during the 1930s (Taylor 1985). This area of study grew slowly until, beginning in the early 1960s, neuroleptics were introduced for treating psychotic and seriously aggressive children. Antidepressants were first widely used with children during the late 1960s, followed by lithium carbonate and minor tranquilizers during the 1970s, and anticonvulsants and beta-blockers during the 1980s for psychiatric disturbances. Today, psychopharmacotherapy is accepted as an integral part of psychiatric inpatient treatment.

Goals

There are two main purposes for using psychiatric medications with school-age inpatients. First, by altering the internal biological forces affecting behavior, the therapeutic use of well-chosen medicines may improve reality testing, observing-ego abilities, and the regulation and modulation of affect. With improvement in these autonomous ego functions, impulse control is increased as well as the capacity to adapt to social reality (Marcus 1990).

The second purpose for psychopharmacotherapy is to assist in behavioral control. Intermittent drug intervention to inhibit aggressive and self-abusive behaviors should be limited to those cases when a specific diagnosis related to the behaviors has been made. Clearly, these two main purposes are not always discrete but are often related.

Pharmacotherapy designed primarily for the control of behavior must be carefully considered prior to its use. First, the clinician must determine the seriousness of the designated behavior. If it is considered more of an annoyance than an actual threat to the patient or others, alternate means of control should be chosen. The clinician should assess whether less invasive techniques might adequately diminish the behavior. Often, rowdiness within the milieu, troublesome group dynamics, low staff-patient ratio, staff conflicts, and peer intimidation, among other factors, can significantly contribute to out-of-control behavior and must be addressed prior to drug usage (Antoinette et al. 1990). Furthermore, the clinician should evaluate whether underlying biological forces are either precipitating or influencing the behaviors targeted for pharmacotherapeutic remediation.

Logistics

Prior to the use of psychotropic medications with hospitalized school-age children, the psychiatrist should meet with both patient and parents to discuss the rationale for the chosen drug, the desired results, how this therapy fits into the larger treatment plan, methods of administration, and potential side effects. Positive and negative reports in the literature, and the physician's own experience using the specific medication, are also discussed. Of course, the final decision regarding medication usage is the parents', not the patient's. If the child disagrees with the recommendation for pharmacotherapy, the parents and clinician should carefully balance the child's reluctance with the medical and psychiatric needs and make a decision accordingly.

Frequently, patients are hospitalized after pharmacotherapy has already begun. It is often the failure of outpatient pharmacotherapy and psychotherapy that leads to subsequent hospitalization. When possible, drug usage should be discontinued shortly after admission so that the child psychiatrist and team can observe the patient in a natural state and can make a more accurate determination as to whether the ongoing usage of medication is required.

PRN Usage

PRN ("as occasion arises") medicine usage to prevent an escalation or prolongation of out-of-control behaviors is generally considered to be acceptable treatment. Nevertheless, very few studies currently available have assessed PRN psychotropic usage and effectiveness. Vitiello et al. (1987) found little correlation between PRN usage and patient diagnosis and neurological status. Although few side effects were noted, effectiveness was questionable. Garrison and colleagues (1990) reported that thioridazine (68.1% of administrations), lorazepam (10.3%), and chlorpromazine (9.6%) were the most frequently used PRN drugs on their unit. These agents were used in response to one-third of the reported unit incidents of aggression, but their usage appeared to be related to the patient's overall agitation rather than in response to a specific mode of aggression. Popper's (1990) recent survey of New England practitioners revealed that diphenhydramine, chlorpromazine, haloperidol, and lorazepam were most frequently used for behavioral control. Forty percent of unit directors surveyed preferred aggressive PRN dosing to ensure quick response, and 10% used repeated small doses, while 50% combined both strategies.

Popper's (1990) discussion of problems associated with PRN usage is relevant. Prior discussion with the child and prior parental consent are often omitted. Parents are rarely told about the lack of research data to support PRN drug usage. Sometimes unit staff members use PRN medications in a threatening way to coerce patients into reasonable behavior. In addition, on-call physicians who do not know the patient often prescribe PRN medication with the hope that unit nursing staff, who do know the patient, are appropriately requesting it.

In our opinion, the use of PRN medications on a children's unit should be avoided. PRN orders are generally written for the convenience of the psychiatrists and nurses, allowing staff to promptly use a medication for an acutely agitated or aggressive child without having to contact the psychiatrist each time. We prefer that the psychiatrist be called in such circumstances. At that point, a single-dose or routinely scheduled medicine should be ordered, if appropriate. Nonmedication interventions should also be considered. PRN orders are often overused and become routine orders by default, without being adequately evaluated. If the psychiatrist is not promptly available to respond to the needs of an acutely agitated child, then this lack of availability must be addressed and should not be obscured by the use of PRN medications. Furthermore, the use of psychotropics to prevent the development of problematic behavior prior to its presentation is inappropriate and should be avoided.

Termination

As part of the inpatient discharge process, the usage of all medicines should be reexamined. Generally, medication should be discontinued 3 to 4 months following symptom-free behavior. This is especially important with public patients who have very limited access to child psychiatry following discharge. Often hospital medication regimes are continued by primary care physicians for unnecessarily extended periods of time following discharge of these patients.

Specific Medications

Antipsychotics

As in adult schizophrenic patients, neuroleptics have become the treatment of choice for prepubertal childhood schizophrenia. However it is somewhat surprising that there are no systematic studies supporting their use in treating childhood psychosis. Anecdotally, neuroleptics appear to be less effective with children than with adults. Antipsychotics are frequently used to treat aggressive and self-abusive behaviors in both mentally retarded and autistic children. Haloperidol has been shown to be superior to placebo in facilitating discrimination learning in autistic patients (Anderson et al. 1984; Campbell and Spencer 1988). Chlorpromazine, mesoridazine, thioridazine, and haloperidol may be useful in managing self-injurious behavior in mentally retarded patients, although there are few studies (Farber 1987). Haloperidol and pimozide are effective in treating the symptoms of Tourette's syndrome (Bruun 1984). Antipsychotics also are frequently used to manage aggressive behaviors secondary to conduct disorder and organic mental disorder (Campbell et al. 1984; Werry and Aman 1975) (see Chapter 13).

Currently there are no available studies describing *optimal* dosage or frequency and route of administration for the various antipsychotics when used to treat the symptom patterns described above. Campbell and Spencer (1988) suggest that a 4-week trial should be sufficient to determine drug efficacy, and that after 4 to 6 months of therapy, the drug should be stopped to determine continued need. Specific dosage depends on the chosen medicine, the individual patient, and the particular symptom pattern. In Popper's (1990) review of standard practices for treating acute agitation, chlorpromazine was administered in 25- to 100-mg doses every $1\frac{1}{2}$ to 2 hours to a maximum dose of 200 to 1,000 mg per 24 hours, while haloperidol was given in 2- to 5-mg increments every 2 hours to a maximal dose of 10 to 20 mg per 24 hours.

Generally, the clinician is well advised to operate more conservatively than the practices noted above when prescribing antipsychotics. Possible short- and long-term side effects of antipsychotics seriously limit their utility in hospital practice. They should only be used in response to particular symptoms (i.e., hallucinations, delusions, out-of-control aggression, self-abuse, and tics) associated with specific diagnoses (i.e., schizophrenia, affective disorder, organic mental disorder, Tourette's syndrome, and some examples of conduct disorder) (see Chapter 13).

The following case example demonstrates the inpatient usage of an appropriate neuroleptic:

Timmy, a 7-year-old, was admitted to our university unit following a suicide attempt and very aggressive behavior provoked by auditory hallucinations. There was an extensive family history of schizophrenia. Shortly after admission, he began to display delusional thinking. He insisted that he was transformed into a werewolf each night at which time he escaped the unit and killed randomly. Each morning he tried to prove the story to child care workers by showing imagined specks of blood on his teeth, changes in the lock on the unit door, etc. In addition, he had been observed during unit quiet time talking aloud as though he were responding to auditory hallucinations. He neither endorsed nor denied that possibility when questioned.

Timmy was begun on 0.5 mg of haloperidol twice per day, which was increased to three times per day during the week following admission. Within a few days the symptoms were no longer evident. He continued on this drug throughout the remainder of his hospitalization without side effects.

Antidepressants

Well-controlled double-blind studies have thus far failed to demonstrate the efficacy of antidepressants in prepubertal depressed children (Campbell and Spencer 1988). Nevertheless, these medications, especially the tricyclic and serotonin reuptake blocking agents, are often empirically prescribed for depressed children. They are also used as a second choice to treat symptoms of attention-deficit hyperactivity disorder (ADHD); both monoamine oxidase (MAO) inhibitors (Zametkin and Rapoport 1987) and the tricyclics (Gittelman-Klein 1987) have shown promise, the latter having been demonstrated to be effective in managing aggression associated with ADHD (Winsberg et al. 1972). Imipramine (Gittelman-Klein and Klein 1971) and desipramine are reportedly effective in the treatment of acute separation-anxiety disorder, as is fluoxetine in the treatment of compulsive symptoms. Tricyclic antidepressants and MAO inhibitors have been shown to enhance the treatment of some eating disorder patients in studies of adult women (Freeman and Hampson 1987; Walsh et al. 1984).

In our experience, desipramine and nortriptyline have been useful in treating children with separation-anxiety disorder. Furthermore, both have helped some of our depressed patients by freeing up affect and thus facilitating other therapies. Desipramine is preferred to imipramine because of the latter's anticholinergic side effects. Fluoxetine has substantially reduced compulsive behaviors in two of our patients with pervasive developmental disorder and one with obsessive-compulsive disorder.

The pharmacokinetics of the tricyclics have been extensively studied (Geller et al. 1985), although, just as with other classes of medicines, specific dosage guidelines await further study. A starting dose of 1 to 1.5 mg/kg per day of imipramine with gradual increases usually leads to a therapeutic level within 2 to 3 weeks (Campbell and Spencer 1988). For our hospital's clinical laboratory, this therapeutic range is 100–200 nanograms/ml for combined imipramine-desipramine levels. Fluoxetine is generally used in a dosage range of 20 to 40 mg per day.

The dietary restrictions necessary with the MAO inhibitors limit their usage. Because of cardiovascular side effects secondary to tricyclic usage (Bartels et al. 1991), as well as recent reports of sudden death in prepubertal children (Biederman 1991; Medical Letter 1990; Riddle et al. 1991), imipramine and desipramine should be used with caution, and all tricyclics should be monitored with serial electrocardiographic tracings. Recent reports offering dosage guidelines for the safe usage of tricyclics are helpful (Schroeder et al. 1989).

Benzodiazepines

The efficacy of benzodiazepines in treating childhood disorders has only recently been studied. Alprazolam has been identified as being particularly effective for the treatment of separation-anxiety disorder (Garfinkel 1990). Because of their effect on Stage 4 sleep, benzodiazepines are useful in treating somnambulism and night terrors (Campbell and Spencer 1988). Also, lorazepam has been reported to relieve acute agitation (Popper 1990).

Alprazolam treatment is usually begun at 0.25 mg once or twice per day, and patients usually respond favorably on 1 mg or less per 24 hours. The usual initial administration of lorazepam for acute agitation is 0.5 mg every 90 minutes to a maximal dose of 3 mg per day (Popper 1990). Both are sometimes used in conjunction with other drugs: the combination of tricyclics and alprazolam to treat separation-anxiety disorder, and lorazepam and an antipsychotic to manage violent aggression. Among the side effects that limit the utility of these agents is the disinhibition of aggression sometimes seen after their usage (Rogers and Waters 1985), especially in patients with organic mental disorder.

Lithium Carbonate

The occurrence of bipolar disorder in childhood is now well accepted, and the efficacy of lithium carbonate in its treatment has been demonstrated in recent studies (DeLong and Aldershof 1987; Stewart et al. 1990). The increasing recognition of this disorder has been associated with an increased usage of lithium in inpatient units. Five of our 300 university unit inpatients since 1984 were diagnosed with bipolar disorder and treated very successfully with lithium carbonate.

Lithium may also be useful in the treatment of aggression in boys with conduct disorder. Recent studies have shown it to be more effective than haloperidol, which was also statistically superior to placebo (Campbell et al. 1984). In another study, Campbell et al. (1972) demonstrated lithium's efficacy with mentally retarded self-abusive children. With severely and profoundly retarded, self-abusive, and aggressive children and adolescents, however, it has been our experience that lithium is most useful in diminishing symptoms secondary to either an underlying affective disorder or an organic mood disorder.

Lithium is administered to children and adults similarly. However, optimal blood levels for treating bipolar disorder and aggression in children have not been established, although levels of 0.6–0.9 meq/L have been reportedly used successfully for aggression and self-injurious behavior (Cooper and Fowlie 1973). After following a total of 196 patients taking lithium for up to 10 years, DeLong and Aldershof (1987) reported no serious side effects (Campbell and Spencer 1988). Nevertheless, this drug needs to be used with caution, especially with younger children. Serial laboratory tests to measure kidney, cardiac, and thyroid function are essential.

Anticonvulsants

Carbamazepine is frequently used to treat behavioral symptoms associated with mental retardation and organic personality disorder, and also to treat the episodic dyscontrol syndrome (Farber 1987). There are anecdotal reports in the literature of its efficacy in treating aggression secondary to conduct disorder, although there are no controlled studies (Stewart et al. 1990). Although carbamazepine has been used successfully as a second-line drug to treat adult bipolar disorder, its efficacy has not been reasonably established for children with bipolar illness, and there is one report of increased aggression associated with its use in this group (Myers and Carrera 1989). Finally, some studies have suggested carbamazepine for the treatment of aggressive behavior in adolescents who have seizure foci (Yudofsky et al. 1987). It has been our experience that carbamazepine can be very helpful in treating episodic dyscontrol, especially in children with organic mental disorder. Its utility in treating aggressive symptoms secondary to conduct disorder, however, is questionable.

Although there are no current standards for the optimal dosage of carbamazepine for out-of-control and aggressive behaviors, anecdotal clinical information suggests a blood level of 8–12 micrograms/ml for an effective trial. A complete blood count with differential is necessary every other week until it is clear that leukopenia has not occurred or is within an acceptable range.

Beta-blockers

Beta-blockers are sometimes used to treat disruptive and aggressive behaviors in children with mental retardation. Propranolol (which has a shorter half-life and acts centrally) and nadolol (which has a longer half-life and acts peripherally) have shown efficacy in managing aggressive symptoms in mentally retarded patients when combined with neuroleptics, allowing the neuroleptics to be used in a lesser dosage (Campbell and Spencer 1988; Ratey et al. 1986). Schreier (1979) reports success with nadolol in the treatment of postencephalitic psychosis in a child. Stewart et al. (1990) indicate that both these drugs have been used effectively in treating episodic dyscontrol and aggressive outbursts in children with conduct disorder (Kuperman and Stewart 1987). We have found beta-blockers to be useful in treating neuroleptic-induced extrapyramidal side effects. In our experience, they are also effective in combination with neuroleptics in managing aggressive outbursts in both mentally retarded and conduct-disordered patients.

There are few dosage and administration guidelines in the literature, however. Because of potential cardiovascular side effects, these agents should be used conservatively. The initial propranolol dose is usually 10 mg twice per day. This is increased slowly while monitoring pulse and blood pressure.

Opiate Antagonists

Both naloxone and naltrexone have been used to treat self-injurious behavior in mentally retarded patients. Following the rationale that self-abuse occurs to stimulate endorphin production, the opiate antagonists are used to block endorphins and thus reduce long-term self-abuse. Several case reports suggest that naloxone shows promise in treating self-injurious behavior. However, this agent must be administered intravenously, clinically limiting its utility. Although naltrexone is administered orally, there are no current studies evaluating its efficacy.

Stimulants

Methylphenidate and dextroamphetamine are the drugs of choice for symptoms of ADHD. The former has been shown to increase academic performance, to improve social behavior, and to have positive influences on the child's relationship with parents and teachers (Douglas et al. 1986), and the effects of dextroamphetamine are similar. Others have suggested that aggression associated with ADHD is positively affected by stimulant usage (Barkley 1979; Stewart et al. 1990). Nevertheless, the use of stimulants continues to be controversial within and outside of child psychiatry.

These drugs are rarely the central part of an inpatient treatment plan, because hyperactivity, in and of itself, does not warrant hospitalization. They are frequently used, however, because of the association of ADHD with aggression, the most frequently noted symptom precipitating psychiatric hospitalization of school-age children. The inpatient dosage schedule is similar to that for outpatients.

Anticholinergics, Antihistamines, and Antimuscarinics

Diphenhydramine and hydroxyzine are frequently used to treat acute agitation in 25- to 50-mg increments every 30 minutes to 2 hours up to a maximal dose of 100–300 mg per 24 hours (Popper 1990). These two drugs (as well as trihexyphenidyl hydrochloride and benztropine mesylate) are also used to treat extrapyramidal side effects secondary to neuroleptic usage. Some physicians prescribe them automatically when prescribing neuroleptics in anticipation of untoward side effects. We think that it is not advisable, however, to give a medication until a need has been demonstrated.

Miscellaneous

The serotonergic antagonist fenfluramine was initially reported to favorably influence intelligence and social interactiveness in autistic children (Ritvo et al. 1983). Later studies, however, have failed to replicate the initial results. Side effects of irritability have been reported.

The antihypertensive clonidine has also shown promise in treating ADHD symptoms (Hunt et al. 1985) as well as some efficacy in decreasing symptoms of Tourette's syndrome. We believe that further studies are necessary before clonidine is regularly used for either ADHD or Tourette's syndrome, especially in view of its tendency to cause hypotension and its unwieldy dosage administration.

The integration of pharmacotherapy with other therapies for specific symptoms and diagnostic clusters is discussed in Chapter 13.

Confounding Issues

Failure to coordinate the goals of specific drug treatment with the overall hospitalization goals leads to a disjointed inpatient therapeutic approach. Both overreliance on pharmacotherapy and its underutilization are examples. Both extremes compromise quality care.

Schowalter's (1989) excellent discussion of the psychodynamics of medication usage highlights the importance of balancing pharmacological and psychotherapeutic approaches to ensure quality care. Achieving this balance is predicated on a number of issues, among them the physician's ability to understand at what point a patient's anxiety and internal biological pressures become detrimental to reasonable interpersonal interaction within the milieu and in the various therapies. At that point medication should be used to modify the forces contributing to or precipitating the untoward behaviors. Other therapies are almost always necessary to continue the resocialization and reeducation process so important to long-term patient improvement (Karasu 1982; Satterfield et al. 1987). In order to achieve this balance for each patient, clinicians must sincerely examine their own views about both psychodynamics and medication. Those who are philosophically predisposed against either medication usage or the notion of psychodynamics must confront their bias, and supplement their training where necessary, to be able to offer their patients reasonable and comprehensive treatment.

In addition, clinicians must strive to understand the meaning to their patients of the drugs that have been prescribed. It is necessary to discuss the pros and cons (i.e., effectiveness and side effects) of prospective medications with the patient and parents. The family's preconceptions about specific drugs and idiosyncratic notions about drug taking should be explored. The development of a therapeutic alliance between the clinician and family is vital to obtain compliance with the pharmacotherapy regimen following hospitalization (Book 1987; Schowalter 1989).

Each of the medications described above potentially causes untoward effects that, if not recognized and appropriately treated, lead to varying degrees of morbidity. Especially pernicious side effects include the following: neuroleptic malignant syndrome and tardive and withdrawal dyskinesias secondary to the usage of neuroleptics; cardiotoxicity associated with the tricyclic antidepressants; hypertensive crisis sometimes seen with MAO inhibitors; thyroid and kidney adverse effects following the usage of lithium carbonate; neutropenia and hematopoietic depression with carbamazepine; and bradycardia following beta-blocker usage. Furthermore, exceeding the accepted dosage of each of these medications has additional consequences.

The coordination of medication management between the physicians and the nursing staff is vital for prompt recognition of untoward side effects and subsequent treatment. The use of rating scales for abnormal movements (e.g., Abnormal Involuntary Movement Scale [AIMS], the Abridged Simpson Scale, the Clinical Global Impressions Scales) at least once per week is mandatory during a period of neuroleptic usage (Campbell and Palij 1985; Campbell and Spencer 1988; Campbell et al. 1984; Simpson et al. 1979). Other procedures such as electrocardiograms, thyroid and kidney function tests, complete blood counts, and monitoring of vital signs should routinely be performed and reviewed depending on the specific drugs being used as well as their dosage and route of administration.

A final area of concern involves the increasingly shortened lengths of stay on inpatient units. As discussed in Chapter 2, length of stay is often determined by pragmatic issues beyond the control of the patient and clinician. Sometimes, the length of stay is altered in such a way that there is not sufficient time for the clinician to fully evaluate the effectiveness of a specific drug or to monitor the development of possible side effects. For example, it often takes 2 to 3 weeks after the inception of tricyclic therapy to determine its efficacy. If a tricyclic is started 10 days following admission, the patient's length of stay would have to be approximately 1 month for an inpatient determination of its utility and possible side effects. The same is true for almost all of the medications used, although the amount of time necessary to determine the effectiveness and safety for each varies according to individual pharmacokinetics. Shortened lengths of stay make communication between the inpatient and posthospitalization clinicians that much more important. The inpatient physician must clearly impart the reasons and symptoms that led to specific drug therapy, the patient's reactions to the therapy during the hospitalization process, the short- and long-term goals for the medication usage, and indications for its termination.

References

Anderson LT, Campbell M, Grega DM, et al: Haloperidol in the treatment of infantile autism: effects on learning and behavioral symptoms. Am J Psychiatry 141:1195–1202, 1984

Antoinette T, Iyengar S, Puig-Antich J: Is locked seclusion necessary for children under the age of 14? Am J Psychiatry 147:1283–1289, 1990

Barkley R: Using stimulant drugs in the classroom. School Psychology Review 8:412–425, 1979

Bartels MG, Varley CK, Mitchell J, et al: Pediatric cardiovascular effects of imipramine and desipramine. J Am Acad Child Adolesc Psychiatry 30:100–103, 1991

Biederman J: Sudden death in children treated with a tricyclic antidepressant. J Am Acad Child Adolesc Psychiatry 30:495–498, 1991

Book H: Some psychodynamics of non-compliance. Can J Psychiatry 32:115–117, 1987

Bruun RD: Gilles de la Tourette's syndrome: an overview of clinical experience. J Am Acad Child Adolesc Psychiatry 23:126–133, 1984

Campbell M, Palij M: Measurement of side effects including tardive dyskinesia. Psychopharmacol Bull 21:1063–1084, 1985

Campbell M, Spencer EK: Psychopharmacology in child and adolescent psychiatry: a review of the past five years. J Am Acad Child Adolesc Psychiatry 27:269–279, 1988

Campbell M, Fish B, Korein J, et al: Lithium and chlorpromazine: a controlled crossover study of hyperactive severely disturbed young children. Journal of Autism and Childhood Schizophrenia 2:234–263, 1972

Campbell M, Small AM, Green WH, et al: Behavioral efficacy of haloperidol and lithium carbonate: a comparison in hospitalized aggressive children with conduct disorder. Arch Gen Psychiatry 41:650–656, 1984

Cooper AF, Fowlie HC: Control of gross self-mutilation with lithium carbonate. Br J Psychiatry 122:370–371, 1973

DeLong GR, Aldershof AL: Long-term experience with lithium treatment in childhood: correlation with clinical diagnosis. J Am Acad Child Adolesc Psychiatry 26:389–394, 1987

Douglas V, Barr R, O'Neill M, et al: Short-term effects of methylphenidate on the cognitive, learning and academic performance of children with attention deficit disorder in the laboratory and the classroom. J Child Psychol Psychiatry 27:191–211, 1986

Farber JM: Psychopharmacology of self-injurious behavior in the mentally retarded. J Am Acad Child Adolesc Psychiatry 26:296–302, 1987

Freeman C, Hampson M: Fluoxetine as a treatment for bulimia nervosa. Int J Obes 3 (suppl):171–177, 1987

Garfinkel B: Treatment of anxiety disorders. Paper presented at Case Conference, Division of Child Psychiatry, Tulane University Medical Center. October 1990

Garrison WT, Ecker B, Friedman M, et al: Aggression and counteraggression during child psychiatric hospitalization. J Am Acad Child Adolesc Psychiatry 29:242–250, 1990

Geller B, Farooki ZQ, Cooper TB, et al: Serial ECG measurements at controlled plasma levels of nortriptyline in depressed children. Am J Psychiatry 142:1095–1097, 1985

Gittelman-Klein R: Pharmacotherapy of childhood hyperactivity: an update, in Psychopharmacology: The Third Generation of Progress. Edited by Meltzer HY. New York, Raven, 1987, pp 1215–1224

Gittelman-Klein R, Klein D: Controlled imipramine treatment of school phobia. Arch Gen Psychiatry 25:204–207, 1971

Hunt RD, Minderaa RB, Cohen DJ: Clonidine benefits children with attention deficit disorder and hyperactivity: report of a double-blind placebo-crossover therapeutic trial. J Am Acad Child Adolesc Psychiatry 24:617–629, 1985

Karasu TB: Psychotherapy and pharmacotherapy: toward an integrative model. Am J Psychiatry 139:1102–1113, 1982

Kuperman S, Stewart MA: Use of propranolol to decrease aggressive outbursts in younger patients. Psychosomatics 28:315–319, 1987

Marcus ER: Integrating psychopharmacotherapy, psychotherapy, and mental structure in the treatment of patients with personality disorders and depression. Psychiatr Clin North Am 13:255–263, 1990

Medical Letter: Sudden death in children treated with a tricyclic antidepressant. Med Lett Drugs Ther 32:53, 1990

Myers WC, Carrera F III: Carbamazepine-induced mania with hypersexuality in a 9-year-old boy. Am J Psychiatry 146:400, 1989

Popper C: PRN medications and chemical restraint. American Academy of Child and Adolescent Psychiatry Newsletter, Summer 1990, pp 7–8

Ratey J, Mikkelsen F, Smith G, et al: Beta-blockers in the severely and profoundly mentally retarded. J Clin Psychopharmacol 6:103–107, 1986

Riddle MA, Nelson JC, Kleinman CS, et al: Sudden death in children receiving Norpramin: a review of three reported cases and commentary. J Am Acad Child Adolesc Psychiatry 30:104–108, 1991

Ritvo ER, Freeman BJ, Geller E, et al: Effects of fenfluramine on 14 outpatients with the syndrome of autism. J Am Acad Child Adolesc Psychiatry 22:549–558, 1983

Rogers R, Waters A: Benzodiazepines and their antagonists: a pharmacological analysis with particular reference to effects on "aggression." Neurosci Biobehav Rev 9:21–35, 1985

Satterfield J, Satterfield B, Schell A: Therapeutic interventions to prevent delinquency in hyperactive boys. J Am Acad Child Adolesc Psychiatry 26:56–64, 1987

Schowalter JE: Psychodynamics and medication. J Am Acad Child Adolesc Psychiatry 28:681–684, 1989

Schreier HA: Use of propranolol in the treatment of postencephalitic psychosis. Am J Psychiatry 136:840–841, 1979

Schroeder JS, Mullin AR, Elliott GR, et al: Cardiovascular effects of desipramine in children. J Am Acad Child Adolesc Psychiatry 28:376–379, 1989

Simpson G, Lee J, Zoubok B, et al: A rating scale for tardive dyskinesia. Psychopharmacology (Berlin) 64:171–179, 1979

Stewart JT, Myers WC, Burket RC, et al: A review of the pharmacotherapy of aggression in children and adolescents. J Am Acad Child Adolesc Psychiatry 29:269–277, 1990

Taylor E: Drug treatment, in Child and Adolescent Psychiatry: Modern Approaches, 2nd Edition. Edited by Rutter M, Hersov L. Oxford, UK, Blackwell Scientific, 1985, pp 780–793

Vitiello B, Riccuiti AJ, Behar D: PRN medications in child state hospital inpatients. J Clin Psychiatry 48:351–354, 1987

Walsh BT, Stewart JW, Roose SP, et al: Treatment of bulimia with phenelzine: a double-blind, placebo-controlled study. Arch Gen Psychiatry 41:1105–1109, 1984

Werry JS, Aman MG: Methylphenidate and haloperidol in children: effects on attention, memory, and activity. Arch Gen Psychiatry 32:790–795, 1975

Winsberg BG, Bialer I, Kupietz S, et al: Effects of imipramine and dextroamphetamine on behavior of neuropsychiatrically impaired children. Am J Psychiatry 128:1425–1431, 1972

Yudofsky SC, Silver JM, Schneider SE: Pharmacologic treatment of aggression. Psychiatric Annals 17:397–406, 1987

Zametkin AJ, Rapoport JL: Noradrenergic hypothesis of attention deficit disorder with hyperactivity: a critical review, in Psychopharmacology: The Third Generation of Progress. Edited by Meltzer HY. New York, Raven, 1987, pp 837–842

Chapter 9

Behavior Therapy

Behavior therapy includes "those treatments that utilize the principles of learning theory and applied aspects of experimental psychology and that are committed to explicit specification of treatment procedures and goals and to the objective evaluation of therapeutic outcomes" (Werry and Wollersheim 1989, p. 2). Yule (1985) adds that behavior therapy is distinguished from other treatment approaches by its commitment to the scientific approach to problem solving. Social-skills training, the newer cognitive-behavioral therapies, and classical and operant conditioning are all examples.

Although behavior therapy techniques have been used in outpatient settings since the time of Pavlov (Skinner 1938; Wolpe and Lazarus 1966), it is not clear when they were first used with inpatients. Stone (1979) has suggested that the current use of behavioral techniques has been an outgrowth of the cultist rituals, hard labor, forced imitation, and coerced responses frequently employed in early residential treatment facilities. In more benign fashion, it is clear that the emergence of the milieu as an important treatment force was accompanied by a systematic inclusion of behavioral techniques into hospital treatment.

Behavior therapy has many uses in contemporary inpatient practice. The coordination and application of specific behavioral techniques contribute strongly to the development and maintenance of the milieu structure. Behavioral programs are used to teach self-help skills such as toileting. The incorporation of behavior modification into social-skills training and parent training programs is well established. In addition, cognitive-behavioral therapy has become an important treatment modality for various symptoms and diagnostic clusters (Mansdorf and Lukens 1987). Advantages of these therapeutic approaches include the control of external circumstances, the delivery of a very clear message about what is expected, and the generalization of the principles learned within the milieu.

Milieu Principles

The use of behavior modification techniques is very important within the milieu (see Table 9–1). Modeling, reinforcement, extinction, shaping, imitation, token reinforcement, response prevention, differential attention, ignoring, and praise have all proven efficacious during hospitalization (Rinn 1978; Yule 1985). The establishment of unit rules and consequences for infractions of the rules, the rewards and responsibilities of the privilege level system, the use of time out, and the use of charts and stickers are a few examples of how the operation of the milieu is dependent on behavioral techniques (see Chapter 12).

The most important elements regarding the use of these techniques are how and when they are applied. Consistency, positive affect, timeliness, and encouragement enhance their effectiveness as reflected in the attitudes and behaviors of child care workers, nursing staff members, and therapists.

Praise and Positive Reinforcement

Praise and *positive reinforcement* are among the most important techniques. Many hospitalized children come from emotionally deprived backgrounds where extremes of criticism and psychological abuse have been inappropriately used to control behavior. Without a positive milieu approach, these children continue to be caught in a cycle of self-defeating behavior and criticism. Even those patients who do not come from emotionally deprived backgrounds need a positive-reinforcement approach because of the amount of negative attention their symptoms and inappropriate behaviors have generated in the past. Praise and positive reinforcement are the technical cornerstones of an effective milieu (see Chapter 12).

Positive reinforcement takes many forms. We agree with Yule's (1985) conclusion that social reinforcers are most effective. A child care worker's enthusiastic response to a specific patient's positive behavior is very important, especially when a good relationship already exists between the two. Other, more tangible reinforcers are also used appropriately on inpatient units. Having patients work toward a goal that, once achieved, is rewarded can be very useful. It is necessary that the team determine which rewards will be used within the milieu. The rewards should be consistent with unit

Table 9–1. Behavioral therapy techniques used in the milieu

Praise and positive reinforcement	Shaping
Modeling and imitation	Ignoring
Cueing and prompting	Negative reinforcement

policy and serve as appropriate responses to patient behaviors (see Chapter 12 for examples).

Modeling and Imitation

Modeling and *imitation* are often used in concert with praise and positive reinforcement to encourage specific behaviors and verbalizations. They enhance the process of desensitization for anxious and phobic children and are especially important on inpatient units for helping children learn how to reasonably manage interpersonal conflict. Staff members verbalize for patients appropriate ways of solving problems and handling disagreements and then have the patients practice these new approaches. Modeling and verbal instruction are used following time out, when child care workers help patients process what behaviors have led to time out and what can be done differently in the future to obtain positive attention and to avoid negative consequences.

Cueing and *prompting* are used as part of imitation and modeling in a stepwise fashion to help the patient build a repertoire of positive behaviors.

Shaping

Shaping is an additional behavioral technique. By successively reinforcing the patient's increasing ability to approximate desired behavior, child care workers and therapists send a clear message about how to develop appropriate behavior. Assessing which behaviors need to be learned, how best to shape them, and how to teach the parents to do the same are key components necessary for the generalization of more positive behaviors and attitudes following discharge (Yule 1985).

Ignoring

Knowing when to *ignore* certain actions can help to substantially reduce symptoms and negative interactional patterns. Parents may unwittingly help to maintain problem behaviors by allowing themselves to be drawn into a negative interaction in a way that reinforces the behaviors. Many behaviors will simply cease if ignored. Teaching the parents which ones should be ignored and when to apply other techniques is an important part of each child's treatment.

Negative Reinforcement

The concept and use of *negative reinforcement* are central to time out, the use of restraints, and other milieu interventions. These interventions must be conducted fairly, and the child should be given an understanding of the factors leading to their application. The use of such a technique in judgmental and angry ways often leads to the reinforcement of the negative behaviors for which the consequences were originally intended. As with all techniques, the therapeutic application of negative reinforcement requires skilled training and ongoing supervision (see Chapter 12).

Self-Help Skills

Developmentally delayed and mentally retarded patients often require specifically designed training to develop adequate eating and toileting skills or to enhance the rudimentary skills already in place. Drabman and colleagues (1978), having reviewed the issues related to the development and implementation of self-feeding and toileting programs, underscore the importance of a precise evaluation of the specific level of need and a practical, efficient plan to attain treatment goals.

An effective self-feeding program begins with an accurate evaluation of the patient's specific abilities (e.g., ability to hold a spoon, ability to pick up food with the spoon, ability to use other utensils, willingness to use utensils) and optimal methods for learning (e.g., imitation, verbal instruction, physical guidance, effective positive and negative reinforcers). As with other therapies, the clinician also assesses the unit's ability to implement specifically chosen approaches. Issues such as patient-staff ratio, clarity of the chosen plan, and availability of staff time must all be considered.

The skills targeted for acquisition should be simply and clearly stated and the chosen reinforcers should include removal of food or physical interruption of the negative behavior (Drabman et al. 1978). In our experience, it is extremely difficult to interrupt the disorganized, hand-to-mouth method of feeding seen in poorly trained, developmentally disabled children without physically interceding, as is seen in the following case example:

> Phillip, a 5-year-old mentally retarded boy who had been reared in a physically abusive and emotionally and socially negligent environment, was admitted because of acute agitation and self-abuse. He had not been taught either self-feeding or toileting skills. He ate by shoving food into his mouth with his hands. However, he showed a capacity to learn by imitation and verbal instruction, especially when offered enthusiastically and with accompanying praise.

> A plan was established to help train the patient to physically hold a spoon, to put food onto the spoon, and to then take the food into his mouth from the spoon. Phillip was initially shown how to hold a spoon in two sessions by the therapist who physically put her hand over his. After this skill was developed, the use of the spoon was introduced during meals. The therapist put her hand over his and showed him how to use the spoon to pick up food. He used his other hand to place food onto the spoon. He was praised for being able to get food onto the spoon and for being able to hold it, and was then encouraged and taught how to eat when the therapist helped him bring the spoon to his mouth. With prompting he succeeded. In the course of the training, however, the plate had to be removed several times because of his tantrum-like behavior in response to frustration. It took 2 to 3 weeks of consistently reinforcing the desired behaviors through praise and food removal before Phillip readily used a spoon.

These same techniques can be used to refine previously developed skills. Everything from training patients to use a knife and fork appropriately to teaching good table manners can be readily accomplished if the goals and the program tenets are simply and clearly stated.

Development of toileting skills is more difficult to facilitate on inpatient units. Drabman and colleagues' (1978) description of the state-of-the-art approach (Foxx and Azrin 1973) includes one-to-one staff attention and the use of two automatic devices wired to signal when wet (moisture-sensitive pants and a plastic bowl device that fits inside the training toilet). In this approach patients are given large amounts of fluid and then seated on the toilet for 20 minutes or until they void. Behavioral techniques are used to teach and encourage the child to recognize the need, to walk to the toilet, to sit on the toilet, and to appropriately use the facilities. These skills are taught in systematic, well-organized sessions employing positive reinforcers.

Social-Skills Training

Behavioral modification techniques are employed to enhance the development and appropriate usage of interactional and interpersonal skills. Rinn and Markle (1979) describe four categories of social skills:

1. Self-expressive skills refer to the ability to accept compliments and to express opinions and feelings.
2. Enhancing skills include the use of praise for others as well as the ability to agree with another's opinions.
3. Assertive skills include reasonably disagreeing with another's opinion, denying unreasonable requests, and the ability to make simple requests.

4. Communication skills denote the child's ability to converse and interpersonal problem solving (Van Hasselt et al. 1979).

Several methods are used to assess individual development of social skills, including patient, parent, and teacher rating scales, sociometric questionnaires, and psychiatric interviews. Recently developed role-play assessment programs to evaluate social competence through inter-rater scoring of child behavior are quite useful (Bornstein et al. 1977; Dodge et al. 1985).

Although useful with all children, social skills training programs are especially effective in treating behavioral problems. Individual and group training have been employed effectively with aggressive adolescent inpatients (Elder et al. 1978), school-age inpatients with conduct disorder (Hansen et al. 1989), and outpatient children with behavioral and attention- deficit difficulties (Rose and LeCroy 1985). Recently, to enhance follow-up results, clinicians have targeted children's social perception, knowledge of social rules, and peer group behavior within training programs (Ladd and Asher 1985).

Kolko and colleagues (1990) have used inpatient skills training groups quite effectively for school-age children with conduct disorder or attention-deficit disorder. Initially they targeted eight behaviors for evaluation and subsequent modification: social involvement, child gaze during interpersonal interactions, understanding of physical space, voice volume and inflection, ability to begin conversations and use compliments, positive assertiveness, ability to respond appropriately to provocation, and appropriate nonaggressive play and sharing. Then, a 15-session group to teach and enhance skills development was compared with a 15-week social activity group involving the use of play, games, and semistructured tasks.

The training group approach included the following therapeutic tenets. Initially, group rules were read. At the beginning of each session, the previous lesson was reviewed, following which the therapist quizzed the patients to determine their understanding and recall of the previous week's material. An introduction of each new skill was followed by a discussion of its importance and instructions describing its components. The therapists determined each patient's level of understanding of the new skill's components before proceeding. Then, the group viewed a videotape in which new situations were role-played correctly and incorrectly. Patients were asked to differentiate the appropriateness of the correct and incorrect approaches to assess their understanding of the lesson. Incorrect discriminations led to a review of the role play. Therapists and patients then role-played the situations within the group and subsequently discussed each role-play situation, at which time constructive feedback was offered. Randomly chosen interactions were videotaped and reviewed by the group for discussion. Inappropriate child interactions were identified and correct alternatives modeled within the group. Points were earned according to patient participation. Generalization of skills was promoted by staff reinforcement of the learned behaviors within the milieu following the group sessions and through the use of stickers and praise. The children who participated in the training group showed significantly greater post-therapy improvements than the children in the social activity group.

Of course, social-skills training is not limited to such elaborate approaches. Continuous training should occur within the milieu. Child care workers, nursing staff, and therapists take every possible opportunity to correct problematic interactions and to teach more appropriate ones. Furthermore, unit activities, occupational therapy, community meetings, and structured time such as meal times and school provide additional opportunities for social-skills training.

Cognitive-Behavioral Therapy

The aproach taken by Kolko's group is essentially an example of cognitive-behavioral therapy, the new behavioral approach that has also shown promise in the treatment of anxiety disorders, attention-deficit disorder, and some examples of conduct disorder (Deblinger et al. 1990; Mansdorf and Lukens 1987; Satterfield et al. 1987). This approach underscores the importance of the intervening cognitive processes in patients' behavior. Therapeutic emphasis is placed on both behavior and thinking.

There are several components of this therapy: active instruction to help find alternate solutions to problems, covert self-instruction (e.g., helping patients to look at their own behavior to determine its meaning), reframing of events, challenging maladaptive beliefs, and encouraging patients to develop more optimistic and reasonable attitudes about distressing situations (Werry and Wollersheim 1989). In short, cognitive-behavioral techniques are used to correct patient misperceptions and misconceptions.

Deblinger and colleagues (1990) described a three-phase treatment group for sexually abused children with posttraumatic stress disorder. In the first phase (two sessions), coping skills were taught to help the child effectively express emotions and manage anxiety. A six-session second phase emphasized gradual exposure to the memories and events related to the abuse while continuing to help the child cope with anxiety. The third phase involved education and training in prevention. In evaluating the program, the authors found significant improvement with regard to internalizing behaviors (i.e., fear and anxiety), externalizing behaviors (i.e., acting out), and depression, as measured on various rating scales.

In another example, Satterfield and colleagues (1987) used cognitive-behavioral techniques as part of a multimodality treatment designed for predelinquent hyperactive boys. Emotional and behavioral symptoms (e.g., anger, depression, lying, fighting) were treated with both cognitive-behavioral techniques and dynamic, interpretive therapy. The children were taught to associate behaviors with consequences through cognitive work, to identify interpersonal triggers of aggressive behavior, and to use socially acceptable behavioral substitutes learned through modeling and role playing. The approach proved quite successful in preventing the development of delinquent behavior.

Other Uses

Behavioral techniques are prominently used in family therapy and parent training programs (Rinn 1978). By directing therapeutic approaches to family interactions that promote and maintain inappropriate behaviors, and by using behavioral techniques to train parents to appropriately reinforce positive behaviors and limit negative ones, therapists have provided important additional mechanisms for the treatment of patient and family problems. These approaches will be discussed more fully in Chapter 11.

Specific behavioral programs and plans have been designed to treat anxiety, depression, mental retardation, autism, tic disorders, stuttering, psychophysiological disorders, oppositional behavior, attention-deficit hyperactivity disorder, academic problems, conduct disorder, substance abuse, anorexia and bulimia, obesity, social isolation, and symptoms secondary to child abuse (Hersen and Van Hasselt 1987). Although primarily designed for outpatient work, most of the established programs are easily incorporated into inpatient treatment plans. Interventions used to manage particular symptoms and diagnostic clusters are discussed in Chapter 13.

Confounding Issues

Two primary factors negatively affecting the use of behavioral principles on inpatient units are the lack of knowledge about how to establish behavioral programs and the lack of necessary coordination to integrate organized behavior therapy into the general milieu. As with other discrete forms of psychiatric therapy, behavior therapy has its own language, assessment procedures, and treatment techniques that differ in substantial ways from traditional individual psychotherapy and pharmacotherapy. For effective use of these methods, the treatment team leader must either have experience with behavior therapy or be able to work closely with clinicians who do have this experience and training in order to ensure the provision of necessary services.

The specific administrative structure used on a school-age unit affects the incorporation of behavioral therapies into the treatment plan. The effective and pervasive use of behavioral techniques within the milieu requires a well-controlled, centrally focused treatment environment with a strong unit or milieu director (see Chapter 15). These techniques cannot be applied to some patients within the milieu and not to others. When that happens, patients feel that they are being treated unfairly and often respond with an underlying intransigence that can mitigate therapeutic gains.

References

Bornstein M, Bellack A, Hersen M: Social skills training for highly aggressive children in an inpatient setting. J Appl Behav Anal 10:113–195, 1977

Deblinger E, McLeer SV, Henry D: Cognitive behavioral treatment for sexually abused children suffering from post-traumatic stress: preliminary findings. J Am Acad Child Adolesc Psychiatry 29:747–752, 1990

Dodge KA, McClaskey CL, Feldman E: Situational approach to the assessment of social competence in children. J Consult Clin Psychol 53:344–353, 1985

Drabman R, Jarvie G, Hammer D: Residential child treatment, in Behavior Therapy in a Psychiatric Setting. Edited by Hersen M, Bellack A. Baltimore, MD, Williams & Wilkins, 1978, pp 219–255

Elder J, Edelstein B, Narick N: Adolescent psychiatric patients: modifying aggressive behavior with social skills training. Behav Modif 3:161–178, 1978

Foxx R, Azrin N: Dry pants: a rapid method of toilet training children. Behaviour Research and Therapy 11:435–442, 1973

Hansen D, St Lawrence J, Christoff K: Group conversational skills training with inpatient children and adolescents: social validation, generalization and maintenance. Behav Modif 13:4–31, 1989

Hersen M, Van Hasselt V: Behavior Therapy With Children and Adolescents: A Clinical Approach. New York, Wiley, 1987

Kolko DJ, Loar LL, Sturnick D: Inpatient social-cognitive skills training groups with conduct disordered and attention deficit disordered children. J Child Psychol Psychiatry 31:737–748, 1990

Ladd G, Asher S: Social skills training and children's relations, in Handbook of Social Skills Training and Research. Edited by L'Abate L, Milan M. New York, Wiley, 1985, pp 219–244

Mansdorf IJ, Lukens E: Cognitive-behavioral psychotherapy for separation anxious children exhibiting school phobia. J Am Acad Child Adolesc Psychiatry 26:222–225, 1987

Rinn RC: Children and behavior disorders, in Behavior Therapy in a Psychiatric Setting. Edited by Hersen M, Bellack A. Baltimore, MD, Williams & Wilkins, 1978, pp 365–395

Rinn RC, Markle A: Modification of skill deficits in children, in Research and Practice in Social Skills Training. Edited by Bellack A, Hersen M. New York, Plenum, 1979, pp 107–130

Rose S, LeCroy C: Improving children's social competence: a multimodal behavioral group approach, in Handbook of Behavioral Group Therapy. Edited by Upper D, Ross S. New York, Plenum, 1985, pp 173–202

Satterfield JH, Satterfield BT, Schell AM: Therapeutic interventions to prevent delinquency in hyperactive boys. J Am Acad Child Adolesc Psychiatry 26:56–64, 1987

Skinner B: The Behavior of Organisms. New York, Appleton-Century-Crofts, 1938

Stone LA: Residential treatment, in Basic Handbook of Child Psychiatry, Vol 3: Therapeutic Interventions. Edited by Harrison SI (JD Noshpitz, Editor-in-Chief). New York, Basic Books, 1979, pp 231–262

Van Hasselt V, Hersen M, Whitehill M, et al: Social skills assessment and training for children: an evaluative review. Behaviour Research and Therapy 17:413–437, 1979

Werry JS, Wollersheim JP: Behavior therapy with children and adolescents: a twenty-year overview. J Am Acad Child Adolesc Psychiatry 28:1–18, 1989

Wolpe J, Lazarus A: Behavior Therapy Techniques: A Guide to the Treatment of Neurosis. New York, Pergamon, 1966

Yule W: Behavioural approaches, in Child and Adolescent Psychiatry: Modern Approaches, 2nd Edition. Edited by Rutter M, Hersov L. Oxford, UK, Blackwell Scientific, 1985, pp 794–808

Chapter 10

Group Dynamics and Therapy

Milieu Group Dynamics

Group dynamics often create psychological undercurrents within the unit that strongly influence the behavior and feelings of individual patients. If these dynamics are not well understood, unit workers can misdirect therapeutic efforts. Instead of positively influencing unit behavior, their interventions either become ineffective or contribute negatively to these psychological undercurrents.

Numerous theorists have written about the underlying dynamics contributing to group process and behavior. Bion (1961, 1967) proposed a theory based on two parallel levels of group functioning: a mature level guided by the stated purpose and function of the group and a regressed level predicated on the individuals' needs to manage feelings pertaining to both leaders and other group members (Shapiro 1989). Group functioning on the regressed level is often responsible for the group's inability to perform its stated tasks.

According to Bion (1961, 1967), three shared unconscious assumptions underlie the regressive mode:

1. The group exists for the satisfaction of dependency needs and wishes.
2. Group settings provide an arena for members to fight with leaders.
3. Members and leaders come together to find someone who can either rescue or save the group.

In short, Bion proposed that group behavior is understandable only when its manifest and unconscious priorities are both considered.

The dynamics implicit in individual psychological development proposed by Mahler and colleagues (1975) have also been used to explain group behavior. Soo (1985) elaborated on Mahler by applying object-relations concepts to phases of small group process. During the initial (autistic) phase, children entering an established group usually isolate themselves for a brief amount of time. Because of the neutral role of the therapist and the holding environment provided for the participants, group members regress psychologically and develop transference ties to the leaders and to the group itself. These ties are similar to those developed during the symbiotic subphase of separation-individuation. Patients want to please group leaders and to have their own dependency needs gratified. As the process continues, conflicts develop between wishes for dependency and independence, leading to disagreements between patients and leaders. Following that, group members develop subgroups and cliques, turning their attention to each other. Subsequent hostile aggression and negative interpersonal behaviors are managed as group members work out their problems and reparative processes take over.

Although both of these paradigms, as well as others (see Garland et al. 1973), have been applied specifically to group therapy, they also describe the underlying dynamics that intermittently develop within any ongoing group brought together for a specific purpose. Theorists essentially say the same things about group process: after a brief withdrawn phase, group members must deal with their own feelings about depending on and separating from the leaders. Following this, they must deal with each other.

These dynamics are not consistently present within the unit milieu, but instead ebb and flow depending upon a number of factors. The patients' ages, developmental levels, and individual dynamics; staff countertransference and differential responses to selected patient behaviors and developmental issues; clinical-administrative matters related to unit size, length of stay, and homogeneity of patient population; and treatment philosophy and types and frequency of therapies—all contribute to underlying dynamics and their effects on unit functioning. Furthermore, the continual admission and discharge of patients complicates the elaboration of dynamics, making it much more difficult to understand and predict psychological undercurrents within the milieu than within a particular therapy group.

One of the major benefits of inpatient treatment is the opportunity for therapeutic intervention resulting from the development and recognition of these dynamics. Because most school-age inpatients have enormous difficulties relating to leaders (i.e., parent figures) and peers, helping them learn to reasonably express dependency wishes, to disagree nonaggressively with authority figures, and to relate to peers without scapegoating and excluding others can have a very positive impact on long-term outcome. A major way of accomplishing the primary goal of milieu therapy (ameliorating the problems with the fit between child and interpersonal environment) is to focus child care worker and therapist attention on the sequential development of each patient's responses to these underlying dynamic currents (see Chapter 12).

Conflict over underlying dependency needs is an often overlooked but very influential inpatient dynamic, especially with preschool children and mentally retarded and developmentally disabled patients. Older children are also vulnerable, however, and frequently act out in response to their own conflicted dependency wishes. Some patients openly express these wishes, asking to be taken for special walks and to be treated in special ways. Others seek attention in negative ways, but the attention that they receive does not help them become more independent. Still others ignore child care workers and struggle against any alliance building. Their own problems with trust must be addressed before they are able to work at establishing relationships.

Conflicts secondary to dependency wishes negatively affect unit functioning when they go unrecognized. This is most likely to happen with older boys whose counterdependent behavior is designed to hide underlying wishes, as illustrated in the following example:

> Three 12-year-old boys who were admitted to the unit during the same week became roommates. Although all three were hospitalized because of aggressive and delinquent behaviors, during the course of the first week each exhibited obvious dependency needs and asked child care workers and therapists for special time and attention. At night, however, their behavior became obstreperous, requiring frequent staff intervention, loss of points, and time out, as well as separation of the patients.
>
> The acting out continued until the conflicts about their underlying dependency needs were understood. Although all of the boys were afraid at night, none asked for staff attention because of each individual's fear that his roommates would make fun of him. They nevertheless unconsciously colluded to get negative staff attention (and security) through their behavior. After these issues were discussed during staffings, and subsequently corroborated by the patients in individual therapy, a series of prebedtime meetings among nursing staff, therapists, and the patients to discuss feelings and alternative ways of getting attention were successful in ameliorating problems.

A second dynamic frequently seen in older school-age patients often underlies group scapegoating and bullying of younger or more vulnerable children. Sometimes groups of older patients pick on younger ones to establish a pecking order among the children. This establishment of psychological dominance over more vulnerable patients serves as both a maladaptive means of dealing with unit authority and a defense against the fear of peer rejection. These peer- and authority-related dynamics can be managed within the milieu and in individual therapy, as well as in short-term dynamic group therapy (see below).

Frequently, aggressive and sexual behaviors within the milieu are influenced, if not actually precipitated, by underlying group dynamics. If this is understood and the individual patient's response to underlying dynamics is considered in the ongoing unit evaluation and treatment planning process, group dynamics can be used in a very positive, therapeutic manner. However, if misinterpreted by staff, underlying dynamics can seriously disrupt the therapeutic process of the milieu, sometimes leading to inappropriate counter-reaction by staff members.

Group Therapy

Activity group therapy was first proposed by Slavson (1943) as a process for the emotional reeducation of school-age children. He used play material and food in a nondirective fashion, rather than discussion, as a means of exploring patient issues (Slavson and Schiffer 1975; Soo 1985). The use of this treatment modality quickly grew and incorporated both psychoanalytic principles during the late 1940s and 1950s and behavioral techniques during the 1960s and 1970s. Groups have been used for both diagnostic (Redl 1966) and treatment purposes (Scheidlinger 1984) in various settings including schools, hospitals, residential facilities, and outpatient clinics (MacLennan 1986).

Typical outpatient and inpatient groups include 1) activities groups, 2) social-skills groups, 3) working groups to organize unit chores, 4) cognitive-behavioral groups, and 5) both short-term and long-term dynamic therapy groups. These groups differ according to anticipated goals, group composition and indications for patient involvement, the use of activities versus discussion, the establishment and implementation of rules and consequences, the methods used to understand and manage dynamics, and the therapist's role. In spite of their accepted usage, however, there have been very few reports of their efficacy in the literature. Dies and Riester's (1986) excellent review of research concerning traditional group therapy lists only six anecdotal reports (Abramson et al. 1979; Adams 1976; Bardill 1977; Clifford and Cross 1980; Rosenberg and Cherbuliez 1979; Trafimow and Pattak 1981). However, there have been several recent well-controlled studies reported in the literature substantiating the efficacy of cognitive-behavioral group therapy, as discussed in Chapter 9.

The traditional type of activity group as described by Slavson is rarely used in current inpatient practice. The changes in patient and family characteristics in the past few decades, as discussed in Chapter 1, have had dramatic effects on inpatient group therapy in that the old parameters are no longer valid. Because of the disruptive acting-out nature of current inpatients, therapists must provide structure during the therapy and must be active in setting limits or either the group will become disorganized and nontherapeutic or group members will physically fight.

Schiffer (1986) has reviewed alterations in the basic methodology of activity group therapy and described a newer form of activity-interview group therapy that includes the following:

1. An active, participatory role on the part of the therapist in contrast to the previously espoused neutral, nonintrusive role
2. A less permissive group climate and the use of direct interventions by the therapist
3. Verbal interpretations of patient behavior intended to underscore motivations, meanings, and consequences of actions as well as alternative ways of behaving
4. Other interventions necessary to limit acting out

In short, the previously accepted dichotomy between activity groups and dynamic groups has little meaning for current inpatient practice because all of the techniques that distinguished these discrete approaches in the past must now be combined into one therapeutic approach to contain and treat difficult inpatients.

Crawford-Brobyn and White's (1986) two-stage therapy group model used to treat outpatient impulse-ridden children illustrates this fairly new combined approach. Because of the aggressive behavior of their selected patients, Crawford-Brobyn and White initially paired the patients in dyads according to similar characteristics and styles before placing them in the group. These therapeutic dyads were "pretaught" particular social skills and learned to be together in the room without leaving or fighting. The group room itself was divided into three distinct areas with craft materials, a table and chairs, and mats and a punching bag. Each session was held for 45 minutes, the last third used for snacks, discussion, and the awarding of stars and positive reinforcers. Rules and consequences were clearly stated and strictly enforced, such as prompt removal from the room for major infractions of the rules. Activities were planned according to each patient's developmental level. To curb aggression within the group, controlled fighting was allowed on the mats. Any boy could stop fighting when overwhelmed by simply stepping off of the mats. This worked well, as the patients felt safe about expressing anger, knowing that therapists would not allow the situation to get out of control. Group results were positive; information obtained from teachers and parents before and after therapy underscored that the gains made by group members were generalized to their postgroup behavior.

This combined activity-interview group therapy approach is especially useful in imparting social skills and in helping improve peer interaction. In addition, short-term, specifically focused activity-interview groups are intermittently used to understand and manage problems within the milieu (see case example below). On long-term units, ongoing groups serve as an important source of data to understand and treat underlying individual patient psychodynamics and psychological issues.

In our inpatient practice we consistently use three group settings. The first, attended by all eight of our university unit patients, meets for 60 minutes daily with one activities therapist and several child care workers. During the first 40 minutes, patients are involved in either a music or an art project requiring peer interaction. During the last third, patients verbally assess their behavior and participation and estimate how many points (toward the unit point level system) they deserve for that session. They get feedback and support from peers and therapists, and points are awarded.

The therapists use currently accepted behavior modification techniques (see Chapter 9), especially positive reinforcement (praise, stickers, points), negative reinforcement (ignoring, verbal reprimand, time out), limit setting (the establishment of rules, intervening during inappropriate behavior), modeling, shaping, and discussion. Therapists judiciously interpret underlying dynamics, particularly as they pertain to motivations for negative behavior, and frequently remind patients of both positive and negative consequences for specific behaviors. Cognitive-behavioral verbal approaches are frequently used during group sessions (see Chapter 9).

A second ongoing group, led by the charge nurse and a child care worker, meets for 30 minutes, twice per week, to discuss community issues, to plan and coordinate patient chores, to decide on the unit menu, to plan outings, and to choose the week's point level system positive reinforcers. Although these groups are focused, therapists take every opportunity, using behavioral techniques as well as dynamic interpretation, to help patients understand their behaviors and to reasonably modify inappropriate interactions.

Finally, we also use ad hoc short-term groups to understand and therapeutically manage specific milieu issues. The following is a description of an activity-interview group used to understand and treat episodes of scapegoating and unit aggression:

> Four 12-year-old boys were selected for an activity-interview group because of their repeated bullying and scapegoating of younger patients on the unit. Six sessions were held over 2 weeks. The co-therapists were very active and used the same behavioral, interpretive, and limit-setting techniques previously described. The stated task was for the group to make a holiday mural for a wall on the unit. Patients were told that completion of the mural within six sessions would be rewarded with an afternoon trip to the zoo.
>
> During the first session, the group was passively resistant and their behavior intermittently very silly, with patients rolling on the floor and making fun of the therapists. This was viewed and interpreted by the therapist as a strug-

gle for control. Alternate ways of disagreeing were offered and consequences for disruptive and verbally assaultive behavior were restated. When the behavior continued, the identified leader was placed on time out (outside of the group), and cognitive-behavioral approaches were used to refocus the three remaining members onto the stated task.

The second session began in a rowdy fashion. The patients were reminded of the time left to complete the task and to earn the reward, and of alternative ways of disagreeing. They then began to plan the mural. However, because of procrastination, this process took the remainder of the session.

The third session started more smoothly than the other two. As the members began to work, it became clear that one had been excluded from the nuclear group. Three boys worked together to make and paint a rainbow while the fourth watched. His comments were ignored, and when he tried to become actively involved, two of the other group members physically stopped him. The therapists observed that this was an illustration of the same underlying dynamics that had contributed to the previous scapegoating and aggression by these patients—that is, by treating the excluded member harshly, the other three hoped magically to avoid the same fate.

During the fourth session, this dynamic was discussed with the patients, emphasizing the defensive nature of their behavior. One leader worked directly with the excluded member, helping him verbally respond to the other three and to reasonably assert himself regarding group membership. Both therapists talked with the four patients about their fear of rejection and their own personal experiences with rejection. The therapists encouraged the reintroduction of the fourth patient into the process via role playing and discussion.

In the fifth session, all four patients worked fairly well on the project, which was completed during the sixth session. Much of the final session involved a discussion of the group process and its relationship to unit functioning.

This particular therapy group was very effective in achieving its stated goals. In addition to completing the mural, the patients' unit behavior changed, with a marked diminution in oppositionalism and aggression. By working with the therapists, the patients developed more trust in both the unit process and the staff. By recognizing and therapeutically managing scapegoating, the therapists assisted the patients in altering previously pathological interactions. Information about the boys' responses to the group dynamics was discussed in team meetings and incorporated into milieu therapy, each patient's individual therapy, and the parent training group.

Confounding Issues

Inpatient group therapy dynamics are not easily contained within the therapy group itself. Because the patients involved in this treatment also live together within the milieu, the dynamics involving authority struggles, attachment and separation, and peer relationships frequently spill over into the milieu, just as the same dynamics generated within the milieu often affect therapy groups. As the previous case example illustrates, this can have both positive and negative effects. The three patients who excluded the fourth from the group task (i.e., making the mural) also excluded him and taunted him on the unit between the third and fourth group sessions. This spillover differentiates outpatient from inpatient group therapy. Inpatient group therapists must communicate daily with child care workers, explaining the therapy process in detail and gathering information about patient behavior between sessions.

A second potential complication concerns the use of group therapy in combination with individual therapy. Issues of confidentiality often arise, especially when the patient's individual therapist is also a co-therapist in the group. While it is sometimes appropriate for the therapist to recall individual therapy issues from the group, it is never appropriate for the therapist to remind the patient of individual therapy issues during the group session. Transference difficulties also frequently arise with this sort of combined approach. Some patients are reluctant to share their individual therapist with other members of the group. Others frequently become agitated and angry when their individual therapist responds more neutrally within the group than the patient would like. Skilled therapists must balance gratification and frustration of the patient's wishes in order to enhance the child's reality-based understanding of the therapist's role.

Of course, there are many benefits in combining individual and group therapy. Using this combined approach with ego-impaired children can help them learn to control more competently the behavioral sequelae of their own primitive defense mechanisms. By working with the child in two different settings, the therapist is in a position to respond more directly to the patient's needs for gratification in individual therapy while confronting maladaptive behaviors within the group. For the higher-functioning child, the process of seeing the therapist operate in different ways within the two settings increases the child's capacity to understand that the therapist is an autonomous individual, thus contributing positively to the child's ego gains. Furthermore, the combination of therapies helps children reality-test their own psychological projections as patients have an opportunity in individual therapy to discuss their perceptions and feelings about what transpires within the group (Bromfield and Pfeifer 1988; Pfeifer and Spinner 1985).

Finally, following the changes in unit dynamics from day to day requires the presence of a medical director or milieu therapist who is very familiar with all of the patients and who spends considerable time on the unit observing individual and group behavior. This monitoring is difficult to accomplish on large units with multiple teams, but is more manageable on units with a centrally focused administrative structure (see Chapter 15). Without effective staff coordination it is difficult to understand dynamic undercurrents because of how readily they are camouflaged and how rapidly they change.

References

Abramson RM, Hoffman L, Johns CA: Play group psychotherapy for early latency-age children on an inpatient psychiatric unit. Int J Group Psychother 29:383–392, 1979

Adams MA: A hospital play program: helping children with serious illness. Am J Orthopsychiatry 46:416–424, 1976

Bardill DR: A behavior-contracting program of group treatment for early adolescents in a residential treatment setting. Int J Group Psychother 27:389–400, 1977

Bion W: Experiences in Groups and Other Papers. London, Tavistock, 1961

Bion W: Second Thoughts. London, Heinemann, 1967

Bromfield R, Pfeifer G: Combining group and individual psychotherapy: impact on the individual treatment experience. J Am Acad Child Adolesc Psychiatry 27:220–225, 1988

Clifford M, Cross T: Group therapy for seriously disturbed boys in residential treatment. Child Welfare 59:560–565, 1980

Crawford-Brobyn J, White A: A two-stage model for group therapy with impulse-ridden latency age children, in Child Group Psychotherapy. Edited by Riester A, Kraft I. Madison, CT, International Universities Press, 1986, pp 123–138

Dies R, Riester A: Research on child group therapy: present status and future directions, in Child Group Psychotherapy. Edited by Riester A, Kraft I. Madison, CT, International Universities Press, 1986, pp 173–222

Garland J, Jones H, Kolodny R: A model for the stages of development in social work groups, in Explorations in Group Work. Edited by Bernstein S. Boston, MA, Milford House, 1973, pp 17–71

MacLennan B: Child group psychotherapy in special settings, in Child Group Psychotherapy. Edited by Riester A, Kraft I. Madison, CT, International Universities Press, 1986, pp 83–102

Mahler M, Pine F, Bergman A: The Psychological Birth of the Human Infant. New York, Basic Books, 1975

Pfeifer G, Spinner D: Combined individual and group psychotherapy with children: an ego developmental perspective. Int J Group Psychother 35:11–35, 1985

Redl F: When We Deal With Children: Selected Writings. New York, Free Press, 1966

Rosenberg J, Cherbuliez T: Inpatient group therapy for older children and pre-adolescents. Int J Group Psychother 29:393–405, 1979

Scheidlinger S: Short-term group psychotherapy for children: an overview. Int J Group Psychother 34:573–585, 1984

Schiffer M: Activity group therapy revisited, in Child Group Psychotherapy. Edited by Riester A, Kraft I. Madison, CT, International Universities Press, 1986, pp 223–262

Shapiro R: Family dynamics and object relations theory: an analytic, group-interpretive approach to family therapy, in Foundations of Object Relations Family Therapy. Edited by Scharff J. Northvale, NJ, Jason Aronson, 1989, pp 225–246

Slavson SR: An Introduction to Group Therapy. New York, The Commonwealth Fund, 1943

Slavson S, Schiffer M: Group Psychotherapies for Children: A Textbook. New York, International Universities Press, 1975

Soo ES: Applications of object relations concepts to children's group psychotherapy. Int J Group Psychother 35:37–47, 1985

Trafimow E, Pattak SI: Group psychotherapy and objectal development in children. Int J Group Psychother 31:193–204, 1981

Chapter 11

Working With Families

Alliance Building

Forming an alliance with parents and family members is vital for positive long-term outcome and is among the first objectives undertaken by the treatment team. There are several compelling reasons supporting this endeavor. First, it is not possible to understand the breadth of the patient's psychopathology or the meaning of the behavior without a thorough evaluation of the family and living environment. Second, affecting substantive change requires the type of parental cooperation predicated on a working alliance between the team and family. For example, research has correlated family involvement with positive outcome on adult inpatient units for schizophrenic patients (Gould and Glick 1967) as well as for adults and children with other psychiatric disorders (Sheehan et al. 1985; Withersty 1977). Third, the treatment of the patient's anxiety secondary to separation from family members during hospitalization and the attendant fear of parental rejection demand close family involvement. Finally, the wish to project blame onto the absent (hospitalized) family member is enhanced by lack of family contact.

Of course, the successful establishment of a working alliance with family members is complicated by several factors (Braiman 1977). Parents are often overwhelmed by feelings of failure at not being able to manage their child at home. These feelings may be expressed in variously disguised forms, depending on basic family strengths and pathology as well as the success of team interventions. Some parents overidealize and then identify with unit staff and therapists with the unconscious hope of exonerating their guilt and shame. Others devalue the care provided in an attempt to prove that they can understand and meet their children's needs better than the unit staff. Some parents search for magical explanations; most feel guilty about their contributions to their child's symptoms and are thus very sensitive to perceived blame. Distress about separation from the hospitalized child and the unconscious fear that the child will not return home are additional potential sources of anxiety that often lead to faultfinding and sometimes to precipitous decisions to remove the patient from the hospital. Removal of the child from the home also forces the parents to relinquish those child-rearing tasks that they may have performed well. When family members realize that hospitalization of the identified patient is not going to provide a cure for the family's problems, they sometimes become increasingly difficult. In short, a variety of resistances potentially result from parental feelings of failure.

One of the advantages of a prehospitalization evaluation is that it gives the clinician a chance to work toward establishing an alliance with the parents before admission. The shock of the actual separation at the time of admission can cause intense psychological conflict in parents, especially when their feelings and behaviors have significantly contributed to the problems precipitating admission. A therapeutic relationship with the clinician that predates this difficult time can be instrumental in helping parents over this hurdle and lessens the likelihood of resistances to the treatment process.

To maximize the development of an alliance, the clinician explains to the parents and family members how the unit and treatment team work (see Chapters 12 and 15). The clinician's expectations for each family member's involvement in the treatment process are discussed (see Chapter 4). In short, information offered early about the structure of the milieu and the treatment process is necessary to help parents develop a sense of involvement and to feel reasonably in control of the process.

The clinician and unit staff use warmth and empathy in their interactions with family members. Especially at first, when parents are most likely to appear defensive and hostile, it is important that staff members understand the reasons for parental provocative behavior and not respond in kind. Even when questions are asked in an accusing fashion, staff members should answer neutrally, responding only to the information sought and not to underlying affect. It is up to the clinician to decide when and how to help parents understand what lies behind their behavior.

The following vignette illustrates a mother's anxiety over the admission of her child and the response of unit personnel:

> Jane, an 8-year-old with mild mental retardation secondary to a chromosomal abnormality, was admitted after outpatient therapy failed to interrupt her oppositionalism and her intermittent but serious physical aggression directed toward her mother. During the admission process, Mrs. B. alternately cried about her daughter's admission and peppered the staff with questions about child care on the unit. She refused to comply with the unit policy regarding telephone contact with her daughter. (Usually, children call par-

ents on Monday, Wednesday, and Friday nights, while parents call children on Tuesday, Thursday, and Sunday nights. Mrs. B. insisted on reversing the order and said she would not limit her calls to five minutes.) She was very critical of the physical surroundings and anxiously asked a male child care worker if he "was allowed to work with female patients at night." Unit staff answered her questions nondefensively, and she was told by team members that we would work around her schedule to make sure that she was appropriately involved in Jane's care. She was reassured that we understood that the symptoms precipitating hospitalization would not remit without her active participation in the treatment process.

On the third day, Jane accidentally tripped, scraping her forehead. When her mother visited the next day, she reacted in a very accusatory way, demanding to know who had hurt her daughter. When the child care worker whom she asked could not immediately offer details about Jane's injury, Mrs. B. became even more agitated, accusing unit staff of not knowing what was happening with the patients and threatening to remove her daughter.

The unit director met with Mrs. B. shortly after her interaction with the child care worker. Specific details were provided about Jane's injury, and Mrs. B. was reassured that staff members were appropriately caring for her daughter. The unit director (also the senior clinician in this case) used the situation as an opportunity to discuss Mrs. B.'s fears about her daughter. Mrs. B. readily admitted that she was concerned that Jane had been physically abused on the unit, stating that the patient's oppositionalism and aggression had been so provocative in the past that Mrs. B. "often had to spank Jane hard to get her to listen." In response to questioning, Mrs. B. stated that she had "left marks on Jane" and that she was worried that Jane's problems were a result of her overly punitive disciplinary practices and that we would discover this and "turn [her] over to child protection." The therapist helped her understand her own guilt about her care of Jane and her projection of blame as a defense against anxiety and shame. When Mrs. B. realized that she was not going to be blamed, she was able to warm up to the unit staff, to appropriately join the treatment process, and to reasonably alter her way of managing Jane's misbehavior.

Parent Training

During the early years of inpatient care for children, parents were excluded from the treatment process. During the 1950s and 1960s they were co-opted as active therapists for their children and became more involved in the inpatient treatment process (Callias 1985). Since then, both parent training and family therapy have become principal components of inpatient treatment plans.

Currently there is a range of theoretical models designed to alter particular child behaviors and symptoms by teaching parents and family members specific child management skills (O'Dell 1974). Most commonly used during hospitalization are parent training groups designed to provide support, information about unit activities, and specific psychoeducational material to facilitate positive parent-child interactions.

Parent training programs provide a cognitive basis for parents to understand their contribution to maladaptive interactional patterns and to develop different, more adaptive ways to respond to their children. Behavioral child management techniques discussed in the group sessions are similar to those used by milieu staff (see Chapters 9 and 12). Parent Effectiveness Training (PET) (Gordon 1978) and Systematic Training for Effective Parenting (STEP) (Dinkmeyer and McKay 1976) or a similarly structured training program (Becker 1971) can provide the didactic foundation for the group.

The program proposed by Patterson and colleagues (Patterson 1974, 1982; Patterson et al. 1967) to help parents therapeutically modify aggressive and deviant behaviors in children serves as an excellent example of parent training. As Yule (1985) points out, the key to the program has been the development of complex, reliable, and valid systems of observing and coding interactions between children and family members within the home setting that need to change in order to significantly diminish the child's aggressive acting out. Parents read programmed texts and are taught to clearly define specific target behaviors in individual and group sessions. They are then assisted in developing appropriate responses to those behaviors within their home. A number of follow-up efficacy studies have shown that Patterson's approach is so successful in reducing aggressive behaviors within the home that it is now considered a necessary component for the treatment of aggressive conduct disorder.

As often happens on established inpatient units, we have designed our own approach to parent training. Each parent attends our ongoing group for eight consecutive sessions (see Table 11–1). Although primarily didactically oriented, group process and individual psychological issues are frequently addressed. Because patients are admitted and discharged according to their needs, parents are continually joining and leaving the

Table 11–1. Unit parent training program

Session			
1	How to play with and listen to children	5	Consequences for infractions of rules
2	How to talk with children	6	Time out
3	How to plan a family outing or activity	7	Parental competence; children's chores
4	Household rules	8	Review and termination

group. This contributes to the out-of-sequence character of the group; namely, group members concurrently deal with different issues, depending on how long they have been in the group. Although potentially confusing, this out-of-sequence character has been used to encourage group "veterans" with 6 to 8 weeks attendance to share thoughts, feelings, and experiences with newer members. This process encourages alliance building and the development of trust among newer members and facilitates the termination process for veterans.

Parents are given homework exercises that correspond to the tasks for each group session (e.g., compiling and discussing rules for the home, planning outings). Group leaders begin each 90-minute session by giving parents the opportunity to discuss their experiences during the week with their children and unit personnel. Each parent is expected to state his or her objectives for the particular session, and group members are encouraged to share experiences pertaining to specific parental problems.

During the first session, the group explores how to play with and listen to children. Leaders assign readings and engage group members in a discussion of how to effectively "mirror" children—that is, to provide reinforcing feedback (Masterson 1988) by responding to their basic needs in a developmentally appropriate fashion. Leaders encourage parents to enjoy time with their children and examine the obstacles that prevent mutually satisfying activities. By maintaining a supportive stance, group leaders strive to build an alliance with parents and to encourage their active participation.

During the second session, members focus on how to talk with and encourage children to verbally share feelings of anxiety and insecurity. Group leaders discuss developmental information specific to each child to help parents understand what they can reasonably expect. Group members are encouraged to share their experiences in positively engaging their own children.

How to plan an enjoyable family outing is the main theme of the third session. Paying attention to the needs of all family members and involving the children in active decision making are emphasized. Other group members offer helpful hints about both the planning and the implementation of outings designed to bring the family together. This session, like the previous two, is designed to stress the importance of spending positive time with children. The leaders underscore the belief that rules and negative reinforcers work effectively only within a positive home atmosphere.

During the fourth session, rules for the household are established. Parents are encouraged and helped to devise a reasonable number of clearly and positively stated rules that serve as guidelines to remind their children about which behaviors are acceptable and expected. During the fifth session, consequences for infractions of the rules are devised and discussed. Overly punitive parental behavior and the use of threats are discouraged.

The group discusses how to use ignoring, redirecting of behaviors, limit setting, and the removal of privileges when applying consequences for misbehavior. Parents discuss their own affective reactions when their children misbehave; the group then focuses on how these parental reactions can both enhance and extinguish patient symptoms.

The use of time out is the central theme of the sixth session. When and how to implement this strategy and the display of parental affect during its implementation are extensively discussed. During the seventh session, the group focuses on developing, maintaining, and increasing competence around these parenting issues. Group members explore the importance of establishing chores for children within the home to help with the development of responsibility. The eighth session is used to review previous issues as well as to terminate from the group.

Family Therapy

Few authors have addressed specific technical issues related to hospital-based family therapy. Lansky (1981) underscored the differences between hospital-based family psychotherapy and outpatient family therapy, raising questions about the application of the outpatient literature to this situation. Nevertheless, Combrinck-Graham's (1990) recent review of family systems theory provides an excellent overview of the field of family therapy and family research.

In our experience, the use of a directive, psychoeducational family therapy approach is the least invasive and most efficient initial therapeutic intervention, after family assessment and alliance-building issues have been addressed (Dalton et al. 1989). With those families for whom psychoeducational family therapy is not sufficient or effective, we use structural and object-relations family therapy techniques. In some instances, elements from all three approaches are used concurrently (see case example below).

Our approach to directive, psychoeducational family therapy is very similar to the approach used in our parenting groups. Therapists work with parents and family members to help them establish the accepted standards of behavior within the home, as well as rules and consequences. Although underlying dynamics are noted, they are only addressed when necessary to refocus family members toward therapeutic objectives.

Often, the directive, psychoeducational approach alone is sufficient with parents of developmentally disabled and psychotic children. Furthermore, this approach is the most important treatment component when working with children with anxiety disorders, affective disorders, and some behavioral disorders (Patterson et al. 1967). (Other techniques are also subsequently used; see case example in Chapter 6.) Some families respond positively, altering ways of behaving that previously precipitated or helped to maintain the presenting complaints. For other families the lack of change becomes most obvious during family visits and therapeutic passes when the patient's problematic behaviors, previously contained on the unit, recur.

When psychoeducational family therapy does not work or is insufficient, we next employ structural family therapy, as well as couples therapy. This intervention is often necessary when parental conflict has led to an overinvolvement by the children in the type of decision making and interpersonal interactions that should be reserved for adults. This dynamic underlies many cases of conduct disorder. Structural therapy is used to help separate the children from the conflict, and subsequent marital therapy is designed to help the parents identify and more appropriately manage their own conflicts.

Structural family therapy (Minuchin 1974) involves a restatement of the presenting problems into interactional terms. The therapist directs statements by parents and children toward each other, facilitating an understanding of how each family member perceives the stated problems. Dysfunctional transactions are exposed and interrupted. Special attention is paid to the family hierarchy and power base. The therapist intervenes when children try to make decisions that are reserved for parents or when the parents abrogate their responsibilities. By helping parents appropriately reassert themselves and by enhancing each family member's understanding of the others' feelings and communications, anxieties and misbehaviors can be significantly reduced.

There are very few guidelines indicating when to use couples therapy, instead of or in combination with family therapy, during the hospitalization of a school-age family member. In our experience couples therapy is indicated when specific parental conflicts are contributing to or precipitating the problems leading to hospitalization. Furthermore, just as with family therapy, there are no studies supporting the use of one particular marital therapy approach over the others.

Object-relations family or couples therapy is often a necessary treatment modality when serious character pathology in one or both parents is responsible for underlying family conflicts. Because of the brevity of most hospitalizations, however, its use is usually not fully implemented until the long-term treatment plan takes effect following discharge.

In object-relations family therapy (Dalton et al. 1989; Glick and Spencer 1985; Slipp 1984), family members' unconscious roles and defense mechanisms are identified. In particular, the nonverbal behavior by family members that delineates their images and expectations of each other is closely examined. The goal of this approach is to help family members understand what they expect from each other, how they communicate this to each other, and how subsequent behaviors (especially the presenting symptoms) are a product of these shrouded communications (Zinner and Shapiro 1989).

The following case illustrates how these various family therapies were combined during the hospitalization of a child from a seriously disturbed family:

> Mark, 10 years of age, was admitted to the hospital with an extensive history of oppositionalism and acute agitation accompanied by threats to hurt himself and family members. His problems began 2 years prior to admission with disruptive behavior in the classroom, frequent fighting and aggressive behavior, refusal to do schoolwork, and failing grades. When his parents confronted him about his school performance, he became oppositional at home with intermittent aggressive outbursts directed toward his mother. The behavior prompting admission followed a school conference that included Mark, his teacher, his parents, the principal, and the school counselor. At this conference his mother became quite agitated and alternately accused the teacher of bias toward her son, her son of malice directed toward her, and her husband of not caring. Later that day Mark was taken to a local emergency room because of threats of self-harm, where, during his interview with the psychiatrist, he impulsively tried to stick the metal portion of his hospital bracelet into an electric socket. He was subsequently referred to us for emergency hospitalization.
>
> During our evaluation, Mark cried, had a very sad affect, and refused to discuss his suicidal ideation, but was otherwise polite and made a modest attempt to cooperate. His father wanted to take him home, insisting that the family could protect him. He promised to return the following day to begin treatment. His mother became upset at that suggestion, accusing her husband of not being involved and her son of being "a little shit." The family agreed to our recommendation that Mark be hospitalized, as we were concerned about the parents' obvious conflict and Mark's ongoing proclivity toward impulsively acting out the destructive parent and family dynamics.
>
> The postadmission evaluation indicated that Mark had a conduct disorder, dysthymic disorder, and developing narcissistic traits. He suffered with intermittent separation anxiety, although his symptoms did not satisfy the criteria for an anxiety disorder. He was psychologically overinvolved with his mother, alternately trying to win her affection (sometimes with infantile behavior, sometimes by acting like her boyfriend) on the one hand, while being oppositional and defiant on the other.
>
> Mark's 9-year-old brother played the role of peacemaker. He was supportive toward Mark and his parents, constantly trying to get each family member to see the other's side. The patient's father was psychologically distant and removed from the family. He worked long hours and, when at home, liked to watch television without being disturbed. He frequently used passive-aggressive behaviors, but intermittently became angry, spanking Mark with a paddle. The patient's mother had a serious narcissistic character disorder,

used splitting, projection, and projective identification as defenses, and continually suffered with low self-esteem and a sense of shame.

In the first session (with parents only) Mark's mother described her over-idealized feelings for her father who had died 2 years earlier and her very negative, devalued feelings about her mother, who she said was critical and nonsupportive. The history of the parental relationship revealed that Mark's parents had drifted apart when the children were preschoolers after his mother had had a hysterectomy. She said that she had subsequently lost her interest in sexual relations. The patient's father then participated in a few extramarital assignations while Mark's mother turned to her sons for ongoing support.

During the second session (entire family present) Mark's mother sat between her two sons while his father positioned himself on a couch on the other side of the room. For most of the session, the mother and siblings chatted happily without much participation by the father, when, toward the end of the session, Mark began to play with his watch in a way that annoyed his mother. She reprimanded him. When he refused to stop, she reached over him to grab the watch. After he resisted, they began to physically wrestle, with both of them rolling off of the couch trying to grab the watch. Mark's mother began to cry and called Mark "a little shit." Mark's brother tried to get Mark to give the watch to his mother, and he tried to get his mother to calm down. Mark's father raised his voice, telling his son to give his mother the watch.

The therapists intervened, asking Mark's mother how she felt about the interaction and why she decided to physically struggle for the watch. She insisted that Mark was being oppositional just to defeat her. Mark refused to respond when asked about his behavior. Mark's father said that he did not know why they struggled. When the therapists suggested that the patient was anxious about the session ending and his parents leaving, Mark began to sob. His behavior was interpreted as an attempt to deal with his own anxiety, to pull his mother into a heated (and passionate) interaction, and to draw his father into the action. Mark's mother was instructed to back away from the fight, to clearly tell Mark what she wanted, and to discuss with her husband an appropriate consequence if Mark refused to comply. Mark's father was engaged by the therapist in a discussion of how he might be more actively and supportively involved. The therapists discussed with Mark's brother his feelings and their perception of how he tried to palliate the situation because of his own anxiety.

During the third family session the therapists explained how the children had been drawn into the parental conflict. Potentially effective behavior modification techniques similar to those used in the parent training group were discussed to help manage specific behaviors used by Mark to control interactions with his mother. The parents worked cooperatively to understand these techniques for future implementation. During the fourth family session, both parents insisted that everything was now better and that delving into the reasons for the family problems was unnecessary. When

> gently pressed, Mark's mother became very angry, started to cry, and asserted that the therapists were trying to sabotage the family's gains. The therapists then pointed out that a lack of understanding about the underlying issues might well lead to a return of Mark's symptoms that originally precipitated his hospitalization.
>
> Between the fourth and fifth sessions, Mark had an overnight pass home that went well until the time for his return to the unit. He became obstinate, refused to cooperate, and had to be physically carried back to the unit by his father, who was very angry. In the fifth session Mark's separation anxiety and fears and subsequent need to be the center of his mother's attention were interpreted as motivations for his behavior. The therapists helped both parents verbalize their feelings about Mark's oppositionalism and helped the mother talk about her feelings of inadequacy and sense of shame when she could not "make Mark do what he was supposed to." This became a springboard for a discussion about her relationship with her mother, whom she felt she could never please. She also talked about how she felt she could not please her husband and that she felt criticized by him. She was able to hear from him, with the therapist's help, that she was sometimes verbally critical of him and their sons. During this session, both therapists were very supportive, paying special attention to the mother's susceptibility to painful feelings and subsequent attempts at projection.
>
> Mark was discharged between that session and the next, on his 22nd hospital day, as he was no longer considered to be at serious risk for harming himself. During the following session the family behavior since discharge and parental reactions to the previous session were reviewed. Although there had been incidents, some of which were poorly handled, the family had managed to maintain Mark within the home without a major recurrence of untoward behaviors.

Additional parent training issues were discussed. The therapists discussed how shame, guilt, and negative feelings about the self potentially affect family functioning and child behavior. The necessity for ongoing therapy, which had been broached by the therapists with the parents previously, was reinforced. A specific referral was made at that time to a local family therapist. His qualifications were discussed. The therapists subsequently met with the new family therapist to discuss family issues and progress. The new family therapist met with the family on a weekly basis for 1 year, helping them to explore their personal and family dynamics.

This case illustrates how various approaches to family therapy must be combined for the treatment of seriously disturbed families of hospitalized school-age children. (While hospitalized, Mark was also treated in individual psychotherapy and in a daily assertiveness training group, and his parents attended the parent training group.) At a 1-year follow-up, Mark was doing fairly well in school and had not had a recurrence of major disruptive behaviors, although he continued to be intermittently oppositional.

Other Family Involvement

To enhance parent training we directly involve both parents in child care work on our university unit. During three to four 2-hour sessions, parents work along with nurses and child care workers, learning to set reasonable limits and to enforce nonaggressive consequences with the patients (their own child and other children). Therapists and nurses teach parents how to apply both less restrictive (e.g., ignoring, redirecting) and more serious (e.g., removal of privileges, time out) consequences. Staff members help parents develop experience with and confidence in the use of these techniques. Parent affect is monitored closely and discussed. The use of positive reinforcers within the milieu is extensively reviewed, and the most effective ways of using charts and stickers are discussed.

Some clinicians advocate hospitalizing both mother and child (Johnson and Savage 1967), while others hospitalize the entire family (Combrinck-Graham et al. 1982). This strategy helps to avert the usual stigmatization of the identified patient as the "sick" individual. Furthermore, the disadvantages implicit in the separation of the child from the family at the point of hospitalization are avoided. By hospitalizing the whole family, the psychological splitting and pathological alignment that have contributed to patient and family problems can be more readily managed. In addition, admitting the entire family sends a clear message that all family members must take some responsibility for the untoward symptoms within the identified patient. Family hospitalizations also provide an opportunity to directly assess the minute-by-minute interactions that promote pathology and can lead to a rapid understanding, and possible treatment, of the underlying problems (Nakhla et al. 1969).

Of course, for this to be successful, the unit and milieu must be capable of meeting the family's needs. There must be sufficient flexibility for parents to attend work and siblings to attend school. Furthermore, special financial arrangements are usually necessary because of the high cost of treating the entire family on inpatient units. Nevertheless, the opportunity to continually observe and therapeutically intervene in family interactional patterns can be a very powerful tool, especially for multiproblem families.

Passes

The main objectives of therapeutic passes are to determine if the patient's progress can be generalized to the home environment and if the parents and family members are learning new ways of dealing with conflict. Because of decreasing lengths of stay and increasing scrutiny of hospital practices by third-party payers, the use of passes for therapeutic purposes has decreased. Nevertheless, we think it is important, especially with children whose symptoms are a product of interpersonal and intrafamily conflict, that patients have at least one therapeutic pass prior to discharge.

Confounding Issues

Coordination of family therapy with other therapies is a complex task that requires effective communication among the treatment team members. Inpatient family therapists must share information with the team to facilitate the ongoing evaluation of the patient and family. This information is used to continually modify the treatment plan as well as each specific therapy approach.

Inpatient family therapy is complicated by the fact that the therapist must often achieve two disparate objectives during each session: informing the parents of patient behavior and progress and exploring underlying family dynamics. This requires a well-established therapeutic alliance with both the child and the parents that must be continually nurtured by the therapist.

Finally, an effective parent training program on the unit is enhanced by a centrally focused unit administrative structure (see Chapter 15) and is potentially impeded by the presence of multiple, poorly coordinated unit treatment teams. In the latter case, each clinical team leader must enthusiastically support the unit parent training program and must use similar technical approaches when working individually with parents in order to ensure the success of this approach.

References

Becker W: Parents Are Teachers. Champaign, IL, Research Press, 1971

Braiman S: The establishment of a therapeutic alliance with parents of psychiatrically hospitalized children. Social Work in Health Care 3:19–27, 1977

Callias M: Group treatments, in Child and Adolescent Psychiatry: Modern Approaches, 2nd Edition. Edited by Rutter M, Hersov L. Oxford, UK, Blackwell Scientific, 1985, pp 871–887

Combrinck-Graham L: Developments in family systems theory and research. J Am Acad Child Adolesc Psychiatry 29:501–512, 1990

Combrinck-Graham L, Gursky E, Brendler J: Hospitalization of single-parent families of disturbed children. Fam Process 21:141–152, 1982

Dalton R, Muller B, Forman M: The psychiatric hospitalization of children: an overview. Child Psychiatry Hum Dev 19:231–244, 1989

Dinkmeyer D, McKay G: Systematic Training for Effective Parenting. Circle Pines, MN, American Guidance Service, 1976

Glick E, Spencer J: Inpatient family therapy: on the boundary between past and present. Fam Process 24:349–352, 1985

Gordon T: PET Parent Effectiveness Training. New York, New American Library, 1978

Gould E, Glick I: The Effects of Family Presence and Brief Family Intervention on Global Outcome for Hospitalized Schizophrenic Patients. New York, International Universities Press, 1967

Johnson DM, Savage MJ: The admission of mother and child: an approach to family therapy. Canadian Psychiatric Association Journal 12:409–411, 1967

Lansky M: Major psychopathology and family therapy, in Family Therapy and Major Psychopathology (Seminars in Psychiatry). Edited by Lansky M. New York, Grune & Stratton, 1981, pp 3–18

Masterson J: The Search for the Real Self. New York, Free Press, 1988

Minuchin S: Families and Family Therapy. Cambridge, MA, Harvard University Press, 1974

Nakhla F, Folkart L, Webster J: Treatment of families as in-patients. Fam Process 8:79–96, 1969

O'Dell S: Training parents in behavior modification: a review. Psychol Bull 81:418–433, 1974

Patterson GR: Interventions for boys with conduct problems: multiple settings, treatments, and criteria. J Consult Clin Psychol 42:471–481, 1974

Patterson GR: Coercive Family Process. Eugene, OR, Castalia, 1982

Patterson GR, Littman R, Bricker W: Assertive behavior in children: a step toward a theory of aggression. Monogr Soc Res Child Dev 32 (no 5, ser no 113), 1967

Sheehan W, Blotcky M, Grace K: Forming an alliance with families of hospitalized children. Residential Group Care and Treatment 30:3–12, 1985

Slipp S: Object Relations: A Dramatic Bridge Between Individual and Family Treatment. Northvale, NJ, Jason Aronson, 1984

Withersty DJ: Family involvement on a psychiatric inpatient service. Am J Psychiatry 134:93–94, 1977

Yule W: Behavioural approaches, in Child and Adolescent Psychiatry: Modern Approaches, 2nd Edition. Edited by Rutter M, Hersov L. Oxford, UK, Blackwell Scientific, 1985, pp 794–808

Zinner J, Shapiro R: Projective identification as a mode of perception and behavior in families of adolescents, in Foundations of Object Relations Family Therapy. Edited by Scharff J. Northvale, NJ, Jason Aronson, 1989, pp 109–126

Chapter 12

Milieu Therapy

The milieu of the child during hospitalization is more than the sum of the various therapeutic modalities that have been described in previous chapters. It is, for the time being, the child's "home," a personal and physical therapeutic environment shared with staff and other patients. The overall purpose of the milieu is to provide the type of care that reinforces the unit treatment philosophy and general goals for hospitalization (see Chapter 2). Not only is it important to evaluate and treat the patient–interpersonal environment mis-fit that originally led to hospitalization, but milieu programs must also direct resources toward enhancing the generalization of hospital gains to postdischarge settings. Rinsley (1971, 1980) has ascribed the following tasks to the therapeutic milieu:

1. Provision of shelter and protection (including interpersonal, pharmacological, and physical modalities) that limit and titrate incidental stimuli, thus minimizing the occurrence of further trauma to the already traumatized ego
2. Appropriate and consistent provision of care, including predictable external controls, to change symptomatic verbal and nonverbal behavior into consensual secondary-process language
3. Provision of opportunities for controlled therapeutic regression with emergence of transference material, which in turn reveals the spectrum of the child's overdetermined coping efforts and responses
4. Provision of opportunities for the detection, recognition, clarification, confrontation, and interpretation of the child's and the family's problematic communications and relationships
5. Promotion of the child's identification with healthy, empathic adult caregivers
6. Use of appropriate peer-group interactions to provide carefully monitored opportunities for enhanced reality testing and for the acquisition of age- and ability-appropriate skills

Milieu structure and staff-patient interactions are vital for the attainment of these aims. The structure, including routines, schedules, assignment of chores, the point level system, reinforcers, and interventions, provides reasonable limit setting and also helps to reduce anxiety and promote competence. Nurturance is given during the course of staff-patient interactions. Therapists, nurses, and child care workers strive to strike a balance between the provision of nurturance and limit setting and thus to provide a developmentally appropriate holding environment for school-age inpatients. Attuning the fit between the child and milieu is dependent on achieving this balance. This double task complicates the milieu process and requires active organization and supervision (Harper and Geraty 1987; Parmelee 1986).

Milieu Structure

Feist and his colleagues (1985) have very nicely summarized the history of milieu therapy. Although Freud originated the concept of the milieu, they credit Harry Stack Sullivan with first stressing the importance of providing a supportive environment for child treatment. In the late 1930s, therapists sought to elucidate individual psychopathology by understanding transference within the milieu (Aichorn 1939). Bettleheim's Orthogenic School coined the term *milieu therapy* and sought to create a therapeutic setting for emotionally disturbed children based on psychoanalytic principles. Conventional rules and demands within the milieu were relaxed to allow for the psychological regression thought to be necessary to counter previously depriving experiences (Bettelheim and Sylvester 1949). Although the components of effective milieu therapy were elaborated during the 1950s (Redl 1959), it was not until the 1960s that they were first used to attune the fit between child and interpersonal environment (see Chapters 2, 4, 5, and 6). The importance of balancing unit structure with nurturance to enhance movement toward treatment objectives was not understood until the mid-1970s (Irwin 1982).

Routine

Schedule. The milieu structure is predicated on each child's *schedule.* There is no idle time during the course of hospitalization as each day is planned hour by hour with explicitly stated staff expectations. The routine allows patients to accurately predict what is going to happen during the day, significantly enhancing their sense of self-control. They are able to think about upcoming activities and, thus, to verbalize wishes and concerns. This provides an opportunity to discuss how to achieve reasonable wishes and avoid potential pitfalls. Subsequent success contributes very positively to overall treatment.

On our unit each day's schedule begins upon awakening. Children are supervised and helped as necessary with bathroom activities. They then wait quietly for breakfast, which follows. Then chores, a community meeting, and daily group therapy precede scheduled school and psychotherapy time. At noon all patients return to the unit to prepare for lunch. Quiet time, out-of-doors activities, afternoon school and psychotherapy sessions, and a supervised homework period follow. Children then prepare for dinner. Supervised nighttime activities include play time, games, television, movies, and family visits. After preparing for bed, patients spend individual time with primary caregivers prior to sleep. Of course, schedules must be flexible enough to include both last-minute changes (i.e., pediatric consultations, psychotherapy time changes, etc.) and predictable, expected changes (e.g., inclusion in a family therapy session).

A copy of each patient's schedule is kept at the nurses' station. The charge nurse (or an appointed designee) coordinates and monitors the day's activities. The overall schedule enables child care workers to interact with patients in a planned fashion and allows the team to effectively implement the treatment plan.

Transitions. *Transitions* to and from unit activities are often associated with overactivity and aggression (Garrison et al. 1990). Transitions are especially difficult for anxious, impulsive, and aggressive children who present with extremes of behavior during these times. Unit staff must recognize how particular patients react during transitions and respond accordingly. Not long after our currently used morning schedule was initiated, we noted that following breakfast there was an increase in acting out and the subsequent use of time out. Unit records revealed that the time between the community meeting and group therapy was particularly disruptive. Our subsequent observations showed that after the patients left the community meeting to line up for off-unit group therapy, those children who were lined up first teased the slower children who were last in line. The teasing led to aggressive acting out. The problem was successfully managed through better supervision, by reminding the patients at the end of the community meeting what behavior is expected of them when they are in line, and by assigning positions in line based on points earned during breakfast, chores, and the community meeting.

Mealtimes. *Mealtimes* provide an excellent opportunity for both therapeutic interactions with the children and the provision of nurturance. Just as during transitions, this can be a time of increased turmoil. Problems with self-help skills, social skills, self-esteem, depression, anxiety, and aggression are often magnified during group meals.

On our unit, children wash before meals, then sit quietly in the hall until all are ready to go to the table. As a group, the eight children and three child care workers take their seats in an orderly fashion after they receive their trays. Time to offer thanks precedes the actual start of the meal. Staff appropriately help those who need it, while encouraging others verbally. Child care workers are active in reinforcing desired behaviors.

Offering a consistently rewarding, calm mealtime environment is the surest way of enhancing patient cooperation. It is important, however, that patients be in control of themselves before they sit at the table. Child care workers intervene verbally with disruptive and physically agitated children and remove those who will not readily be calmed. After children are removed, staff help them return to the group as quickly as possible. If unable to rejoin the group after 5 to 10 minutes, the child finishes his or her meal in supervised isolation. Children are encouraged to eat at least half of their food. Control battles are avoided by staff members; children are never threatened or ridiculed. If after 30 minutes the child has not complied and does not have a plausible reason for the behavior, the food is removed and a consequence is applied (e.g., not earning level system points for that activity). Chronic problems are discussed in staffings for subsequent treatment planning. At the end of the meal, the patients and staff clean up and leave the table together.

Patients with special self-help problems (e.g., pervasive developmental disorder, organic mental disorder) are often seated at an adjacent table with a staff member who supervises and teaches necessary skills (see Chapter 9). Anorexic patients eat with the group and are encouraged in the same way as other children. Overemphasis on pathological eating habits is avoided. Overeating is managed according to individual treatment plans.

Bedtime. Children are especially psychologically vulnerable at *bedtime.* Underlying fears and feelings of insecurity rise to the surface, precipitating anxiety and somatization symptoms, oppositionalism, and psychomotor agitation. Patients with authority and behavioral problems sometimes disrupt the bedtime process in an attempt to gain the upper hand. The case example of the three boys who acted out before bedtime in Chapter 10 illustrates this and also shows to what extent unit workers must intervene to regain control once lost.

Children's nighttime vulnerabilities also serve as an opportunity for therapeutic interactions between staff and patients. Fear and feelings of insecurity lead some children to more readily reach out for adult support. Strong alliances are formed when child care workers help children manage fear at bedtime. These supportive interactions help patients develop trust in the unit process and encourage their active participation in the implementation of the treatment plan.

Because they are less well psychologically defended at bedtime, school-age inpatients often verbally allude to underlying conflicts. When pieced together with other patient data, these allusions provide a clearer understanding about the patient's own experiences and psychological reactions. Child care workers communicate this information to therapists who use it for ongoing modification of the treatment plan.

A predictable bedtime routine facilitates this process. Generally, our patients have a light snack prior to bath time. Patients are in bed by 8:30 P.M. on weeknights. Staff members spend time with each patient individually. Bedtime activities between staff and patients vary according to the developmental level and the individual patient need. Reading a story, telling a story, prayers, and talking about the day assist in tension relief and preparation for sleep. When necessary, staff monitor patient rooms to ensure compliance with rules.

Patients are checked throughout the night. Enuretic patients are awakened and assisted in changing the sheets, taking a shower, and returning to bed.

The transition from the bed into the day can be difficult. The desire to remain in a comfortable bed compels some children to resist the process. Each morning unit staff must reestablish the continuously building alliance between patient and environment. A positive attitude and genuine enthusiasm from staff help convince children to get up and start the day.

Morning routine. The *morning routine* itself is fairly simple. The children are awakened around 7:00 A.M. and given a few minutes to collect themselves before morning hygiene and bathroom activities. They then dress and wait in the community room for breakfast while watching television. Following breakfast, they make their beds and clean their rooms.

The level of staff assistance depends on patient need. Developmentally immature patients are physically helped in whichever ways are necessary, while oppositional, difficult children are treated supportively, encouraged to earn their points, and given the amount of space necessary to help them with the morning transition. Structure is provided for disorganized children. Bathroom activity is monitored closely, especially if two or more children occupy the facilities simultaneously.

Quiet time. It is important to include *quiet time* in the daily schedule. Besides the opportunity for rest, it affords each child time to be alone. Preschoolers generally require more than one rest period during the day. Younger school-age children often sleep during quiet time, while older children listen to radios, read, or play quietly with toys.

Chores

Patients are expected to perform daily chores within the milieu. Following breakfast, they return to their rooms to make their beds and to straighten the area for which they are responsible. They participate in various assigned tasks including vacuuming, doing laundry, cleaning, and straightening the dayroom, cleaning the dining area, and emptying the waste baskets, among others. Child care workers assist the patients in completing these assigned tasks.

The main purpose for these chores is to impart a sense of responsibility to the children about taking care of themselves. These goal-directed activities help organize patients and, much like quiet time, indirectly assert staff control and organization within the milieu. Furthermore, chores teach children how to work together in activities that are not immediately gratifying. Finally, they provide an additional arena for staff members to help patients and thus to heighten alliance building.

Positive Reinforcers

As stated in Chapter 9, *social reinforcers* are clearly the most effective form of positive reinforcement. Child care workers' enthusiastic responses to patient behavior are very important, especially when a positive relationship already exists. This developing alliance helps patients willingly comply with the unit routine and rules because of their wish to please the primary caregiver. In addition, charts and stickers are used to build patient support and enthusiasm for difficult tasks. This system is especially important with developmentally delayed and immature patients, but because it provides positive proof of child success, it is readily accepted by most school-age inpatients.

Cut-out cartoon character *stickers* with pleasing smells are offered when patients can complete difficult tasks. Cooperation with blood-drawing, maintenance of reasonable affect by disgruntled patients during activities, and particularly well-done chores are all examples of patient behaviors reinforced with stickers. Prior to and during these activities, staff verbally encourage patients by reminding them of these tangible rewards.

Charts are used to positively encourage and reinforce patient behavior in ongoing tasks. A typical example within both the milieu and the home is their use in the management of nonorganic enuresis. When concurrently used with other behavioral management techniques (e.g., awakening the child, assisting in showering and cleaning bed linen) and psychotherapies, charts have been successfully used in our unit to significantly diminish enuresis in about 80% of the cases.

The child and primary caregiver make a chart with daily entries covering 1 week. This chart is maintained in the patient's room, and the caregiver and patient meet together each morning to discuss the previous night. If the patient has remained dry, a star is placed on the chart and an additional, predetermined positive reinforcer is offered. When the patient has several dry nights in a row, more desirable reinforcers are offered, but over longer periods of time (e.g., for two or three dry nights in a row instead of for a single dry night). Throughout, the child care worker displays a very positive attitude. Enuretic nights are managed supportively so that blame and shame are avoided.

A *point-privilege system* that positively reinforces cooperation with the unit schedule and activities while negatively reinforcing inappropriate behaviors can be very important in teaching and maintaining control on the unit. When the system is applied to daily unit situations requiring predictable interactional patterns (e.g., mealtimes, community meetings, school, chores), the child's entire day becomes a compilation of therapeutic experiences (Dalton et al. 1989).

A variety of point-privilege systems are currently in use on school-age inpatient units. Some are elaborate, involving the assignment of points for behavior during segments of time. The points are recorded on cards kept by patients and signed at least hourly by staff members. Other, simpler systems assign points for specific activities. The complexity of the chosen system depends on specific unit goals and objectives, patient characteristics (e.g., number of patients, types of patients), and the unit's ability to monitor the assignment and collation of points. A description of our university unit point system follows (also see Table 12–1).

A maximum of two points is offered for compliance with wake up and morning routine procedures. Children are expected to voluntarily get out of bed, get dressed, wash, make their beds, and wait quietly until breakfast. Two points are offered for each meal, one for appropriately sitting at the table and behaving and the other for eating at least half of the meal. Two points are offered for chores, one for attitude and the other for compli-

Table 12–1. Unit point system

Scheduled activity	Maximum points awarded
Wake-up, morning routine	2
Mealtimes	2
Chores	2
Activity group therapy	4
School	10
Quiet time	2
Outings, evening activities	2

ance. Four points are possible for daily activities group therapy. One is offered for behavior going to and coming from the activity, one is offered for cooperation with peers, and two are offered for compliance with and participation in the activity itself. There are 10 potential points for school attendance, two each for performance, behavior, cooperation with the homework periods, behavior going to and coming from school, and general attitude. Two points are offered for quiet time (one for playing quietly and the other for remaining in the bedroom). Finally, two points are offered for various unit activities such as outings and evening activities.

After each activity, the points are recorded on a chart in the nurses' station that can be viewed by all patients. How the patients are informed about the rewarded points is important. Several minutes are set aside at the end of each activity for staff and patients to discuss point allotment. For example, following daily activities group therapy, 15 minutes are set aside for the group leader to talk with each patient about point assignment. Patients talk about their own behavior and how many points they think they deserve. Then staff members discuss patient behavior and assign actual points. This process is as important as the actual points.

Although the point-privilege system in itself is positively reinforcing, the points are used to earn various privileges. Each night, points are tabulated for the 24-hour period starting with the previous night's dinner to determine the type of snack the patient has earned. Those who have attained 90% of potential points are offered a special snack, while those with fewer points are offered graham crackers. The Friday afternoon outing (e.g., to the zoo, to the Children's Museum, to the Nature Center) must be earned by achieving 90% of potential points from Thursday to Thursday. Patients participate in the Tuesday night auction of small items (e.g., T-shirts, pencils, small toys) by using earned points during the week. Attendance at other special events often requires a predetermined number of points.

On some units, points are necessary for movement from one privilege level to another. Typically there are four levels, each successive one requiring increased patient responsibility and more adaptive behavior, but offering greater privileges and, usually, more freedom. On other units, levels are determined during staff meetings based on a consensus view of each patient's ability to satisfy level criteria. *Privilege level systems* are most useful on long-term units and work best when objective criteria necessary for level advancement are used and clearly explained to the patients.

Rules

Unit rules play a very important role in the functioning of the milieu. They clearly state to both patients and staff what is expected regarding patient behavior. Milieu interventions are used in response to noncompliance with stated rules. Because they specifically define behavioral limits, rules and their application are as vital to milieu structure as the daily schedule.

There are two basic types of rules: those explicitly stated at the time of admission, and those that are implicitly understood although not necessarily verbalized. The stated rules are presented during the admissions process in a positive fashion as child care workers are sensitive to patient reaction and encourage a discussion of the purpose of unit rules. Consequences for infractions are not elaborated initially, but staff members make it clear that patients are expected to comply. Premature statements of consequences invite resistance in those patients with oppositional, conduct, and borderline disorders.

Our unit rules, which are posted on the door of the nurses' station, are fairly simple. They are written and displayed to invite frequent inspection. They include

1. Participate positively in unit activities and the daily schedule.
2. Listen to unit staff.
3. Eat in the dining area only.
4. Get permission before opening the refrigerator.
5. After awakening, stay in your bedroom until morning report is over.
6. Do not hit, shove, push, run in the unit, call anyone names, climb on the furniture, go into the nurses' station, or take the art off the wall.

Of course, there are prohibited behaviors that are not discussed during the admissions process. Unless circumstances warrant it, staff assume that patients understand that sexual acting out, destructive behavior, running away, stealing, and lying are against the rules. Stating these without cause is somewhat provocative, but if children ask, staff clearly explain and discuss the prohibition of these activities.

Milieu Interventions

Milieu interventions are used to ensure compliance with milieu rules and to help interrupt the pattern of inappropriate behaviors that initially precipitated hospitalization. Wherry (1986) notes that milieu interventions should not be used as punishment, for the convenience of the staff, in response to inappropriate behaviors that could be managed otherwise, or to prevent runaway behavior.

There are at least eight nonpharmacological counteraggressive procedures available to provide necessary correction and containment within the milieu (see Table 12–2). Particular indications and contraindications for each are presented in Chapter 13, in which specific clinical problems are discussed.

Ignoring. As noted in Chapter 9, *ignoring* certain inappropriate behaviors can substantially reduce negative interactional patterns. When used therapeutically, ignoring of inappropriate behavior serves as the least invasive active intervention. It is particularly effective with inappropriate attention-seeking behavior.

Verbal correction. *Verbal correction* is especially useful with interpersonal difficulties, escalating agitation, and sexualized behavior. As discussed in Chapter 9, modeling, imitation, and shaping are important behavioral techniques enhancing this intervention. Staff often intervene by stopping the action before interpersonal conflict leads to physical aggression. They help patients understand why the interaction is becoming heated, how to resolve the conflict peacefully, and what the consequences are for both positive and negative resolutions.

Removal. Patients are *removed from the situation* to help contain potentially explosive and destructive behavior, to decrease extraneous stimuli, and to assist the child in gaining self-mastery and self-control. When removed, children are directed to other activities after verbal intervention by staff members. They are closely monitored in the new situation until it is clear that they have calmed down and can participate in the activity reasonably.

Time out. *Time out* is used in response to a flagrant violation of the rules to let the child clearly know that a particular behavior is inappropriate and to provide an opportunity to subsequently process the incident. As Gallagher and colleagues (1988) have pointed out, there are several ways to apply this intervention. On our unit, time out is taken in a corner of the hallway opposite the nurses' station. Children sit quietly for 5 minutes, after which they process with a child care worker the circumstances leading to the use of time out. When children talk or refuse to otherwise comply with the procedures, the time clock is started over. Some units do not use a predetermined amount of time, but insist that children remain on time out until their behavior has improved. Jones et al. (1990) report that the average time-out

Table 12–2. Counteraggressive milieu interventions

Ignoring	Physical restraints
Verbal correction	Isolation
Removal	Seclusion
Time out	Mechanical restraints

duration on their unit was 16.5 minutes, with 0.2% of the total number of time outs exceeding 1 hour.

As discussed below, the frequency of use for this procedure depends on a number of patient, staff, and setting factors. In the same study, Jones and his colleagues (1990) reported that only one-third of their patients required time out. It has been our experience on both our university and state hospital units, however, that a large majority of inpatients require at least one time out during the course of their hospitalization.

Physical restraint. The child who refuses time out is physically held by a caregiver until able to comply. Younger patients are *physically restrained* in a bear hug with their arms crossed in the front and held firmly from behind by a child care worker. Older patients and those for whom this procedure is inappropriate (e.g., sexually provocative patients) are positioned on the floor where staff hold their wrists (behind the back) and ankles. Child care workers apply these limits without patient injury, in an affectively neutral fashion. Patients are informed that they will be released once they are able to comply with the time-out procedures. Garrison and colleagues (1990) note that the mean duration for this type of physical restraint is about 5 minutes, although patients with conduct disorders and problematic characterological traits frequently require extensive periods of holding, especially when time out is first applied.

Isolation. Patients are *isolated* when they are removed to their room either with or without a child care worker. On some units children must sit on their beds with one toy or one book for extended periods of time. On other units, children are confined within a square drawn on the floor. The decision to use supervision depends on the specific goals for this intervention as well as patient need. Isolation is used primarily to help diminish external stimuli that are precipitating or seriously contributing to misbehavior.

Seclusion. *Seclusion* is the confinement of patients in a specially designed room that is used for this purpose only. Like isolation, seclusion is used to decrease external stimuli. In addition, however, it can therapeutically contain destructive, violent behavior. Specific indications for locking the door are detailed in Chapter 13.

Millstein and Cotton (1990) report that 60% of their inpatients required use of seclusion at least once during hospitalization. The episodes lasted for an average of 15 minutes. Their results conflict with those of Joshi et al. (1988), who showed that the frequency of time spent in the quiet room decreased significantly over time during the hospitalization. In Garrison et al.'s (1990) experience, older patients received longer periods of confinement than younger ones.

Mechanical restraints. Hand *mechanical restraints* (i.e., waist-belt restraints) should exclusively be used to diminish self-injurious behavior. Patients must be carefully supervised during this procedure because of their subsequent vulnerability. They often have trouble maintaining balance and cannot defend themselves against hostile action.

Five-way restraints are applied in response to out-of-control, destructive rage that cannot be otherwise contained. Children are placed on a bed face up. Their wrists and ankles are tied down, and a large leather strap binds the abdominal region to the bed. Garrison and colleagues (1990) noted that the mean duration for the use of mechanical restraints on their unit is 103.8 minutes (SD = 56.6), with a median of 90 minutes.

In addition, some units use a procedure called "lock down" or "shut down," a milieu intervention in which all patients are restricted to the unit, regardless of privilege level and individual ability to tolerate less restrictiveness. This consequence is imposed when the unit director wants a particular (patient) group response to a misdeed committed by one or a small group of patients—for example, when all patients are restricted to the unit until a missing item considered to be stolen is returned. The rationale is that the peer group should pressure the offending individuals to take responsibility for their actions and, thus, to create a more positive milieu.

We disagree with and discourage the use of "lock down" for two primary reasons. First, it inappropriately implies that all patients are responsible for the misdeed, thus projecting blame onto children who have been repeatedly traumatized in the past through similar means in their own pathological families. Second, the psychological pressure created by this staff reaction can be very disruptive within the milieu and gives the false impression that the patients rather than the staff should be in control of important unit decisions.

Several factors influence the use of milieu interventions. Most important among them is the chosen milieu philosophy. Some units, including our university unit, do not have seclusion rooms and do not use mechanical restraints. Others use the gamut of intervention procedures described above. As Wilson and Soth (1986) point out, the choice to allow the use of seclusion and restraints itself leads to their usage. Whether the unit decision to allow or not to allow the most restrictive interventions limits the type of patients that can be appropriately treated has not yet been addressed in the literature. It has been our experience, however, that large 11- and 12-year-old boys who are chronically out of control and destructive during hospitalization must be intermittently treated with seclusion or else the effects of their behavior on staff and other patients can become so deleterious as to render the milieu nontherapeutic.

Several investigators have elaborated patient, staff, and environmental factors associated with the use of milieu interventions. Garrison and colleagues (1990) found an especially close relationship between assaultive behavior toward staff, especially females, and the use of mechanical restraints. Jones et al. (1990) related the use of time out to age and gender. Younger children, especially boys, were more likely to be treated with this intervention on their unit.

Wherry (1986) reviewed the literature relating adult, adolescent, and school-age patient diagnoses to seclusion usage and found conflicting accounts. Schizophrenia (Binder 1979), borderline personality disorder (Erickson and Realmuto 1983), and affective disorders (Gerlock and Solomons 1983) were associated with increased use of this intervention in some studies, while psychosis (Phillips and Nasr 1983) and diagnosis in general (Soloff and Turner 1981) were found to be unrelated in other studies. Millstein and Cotton (1990) found that increasing age was associated with greater use of seclusion. They strongly concluded that the preadmission level of a patient's coping strategies was predictive of later seclusion in that children who coped with stress prior to hospitalization by using suicidal and assaultive behavior were more likely to require seclusion when hospitalized. Furthermore, studies have related the use of seclusion to staffing pattern, staff attitude, evening and night nursing shifts (Wherry 1986), times of minimal milieu programming, and overly stimulating and therapeutically demanding unit times (Millstein and Cotton 1990).

These milieu interventions are most effective when they are included in the treatment plans of particular patients. Which symptom patterns lead to specific levels of intervention in individual patients is discussed by team members in staffings and patient conferences so that child care workers know in advance what is expected. This helps reduce the potential for staff overreaction and emphasizes the importance of overall treatment goals and strategies for long-term patient improvement. Furthermore, each patient incident leading to isolation, seclusion, or the use of restraints should be subsequently reviewed by the treatment team to determine the need for the intervention as well as its short-term effectiveness. Treatment teams must be willing to change or augment therapeutic strategies according to patient response to chosen interventions. Doctor's orders are necessary for each use of seclusion and restraints. The procedures used must conform to written unit policy and accreditation guidelines.

Studies have reported conflicting results following the use of seclusion. Wherry (1986) has listed 16 patient feelings experienced during seclusion, only two of which (feelings of calm and safety) reflect desired outcome. Gutheil (1978) and Joshi et al. (1988), on the other hand, suggest that restrictive interventions can be very positive. The latter investigators noted that 92% of the children placed in their quiet room were calm at the end of their seclusion and that 79% were able to rejoin activities from which they had been removed. Only 7% of their patients expressed anger and subsequent feelings of being victimized following the use of this intervention. Antoinette and colleagues (1990) found that the implementation of an unlocked, rather than locked, seclusion policy on their unit led to an increase in the use of tranquilizing and other psychiatric medications.

Although researchers have begun to look in earnest at the use of counteraggressive treatment techniques in response to patient aggression, current studies need to be expanded in two primary ways before definite conclusions can be drawn about the utility of these procedures. First, units with different milieu philosophies (and thus different levels of intervention) must be studied concurrently while controlling for patient and staff characteristics. This calls for quite a bit of coordination among institutions as well as for advanced developments in quantifying patient behavior and patient-staff interactions. Second, well-designed long-term efficacy studies (see Chapter 3) need to include counteraggressive techniques among hospital treatment variables when assessing outcome before definite conclusions can be drawn about the long-term efficacy of seclusion and the use of restraints.

Activities

Daily supervised *recreation* must be provided to inpatients. After a brief, organized exercise period, children have at least 1 hour of free play. Sometimes staff assist in forming teams, while at other times children play by themselves, in pairs or in small groups. This is to be differentiated from recreation therapy, which has specific goals and treatment approaches. An example of the latter is an organized baseball game in which staff help children learn to play together cooperatively, to establish and follow rules, and to deal with competition and loss, as well as to develop athletic skills.

Music and *art* enrich milieu programs. Activities incorporating both are central to the group therapy discussed in Chapter 10. Of course, clinicians commonly use patient drawings for evaluation and therapy purposes. We have used music therapy in the treatment of developmentally disabled and organically impaired children to assist in relationship and alliance building. Because most school-age children can participate in art and music in a relatively conflict-free manner, these activities heighten patient acceptance and participation within the unit program.

Age-appropriate *board games, toys,* and *card games* are used by staff to engage children in enjoyable, fun activities. Just as with the baseball example used above, both board games and card games can be used to teach social skills during interactive and competitive situations. They are especially useful in helping children deal with sudden narcissistic injury. For example, through these games, staff members are afforded the opportunity to work with children who lose their tempers when they do not win or when they do not get what they want. Staff develop strategies to increase frustration tolerance, to help patients accept defeat, and to impart the skills necessary to compete well.

Outings

Unit outings work best when they are used for educational purposes or as positive reinforcement for the point-privilege system. Of course, safety must be considered first. An adequate number of staff must accompany the children. Those patients who cannot be counted on to behave appropriately, or at least predictably, should not be included. The chosen activities must be appropriate for the group. Just like art and music, outings enrich the milieu experience and can enhance patient participation.

Education

From time to time, educational programs are used within the milieu to impart knowledge or data to groups of children. Sex education is sometimes necessary as part of the larger unit effort to manage inappropriate sexual behavior. On our university unit we recently held daily classes teaching American sign language to patients and staff following the admission of a hearing-impaired child. Information about drugs and drug taking is often included in educational sessions. Whatever information is to be imparted or discussed, these educational programs are approached in an organized fashion with stated goals and objectives. The formal school program for the unit is discussed in Chapter 14.

Physical Environment

The physical characteristics of the unit influence patient progress. Unit size and patient capacity are important variables. Larger units treating large numbers of patients require increased coordination and communication to therapeutically care for patients. Smaller units with fewer patients usually provide a more clinically favorable staff-patient ratio. Whether the unit is open (unlocked), partially open, or closed has an impact on admission criteria, treatment philosophy, and the milieu therapy program.

The unit configuration also has an impact. Areas inaccessible to the nurses' station at night can contribute to patient anxiety and insecurity. Long halls invite running, especially by hyperactive patients. Hidden areas make supervision of patient behavior more difficult. Patients do need private time and private space, however, which units must be able to provide, especially if treating children for extended periods of time.

Access to outside recreation is essential. This can provide problems for units housed in inner-city high-rise hospitals. Our own downtown university unit has had to creatively carve out space for bicycle riding, basketball, and volleyball on a screened-in portion of the hospital roof. Developmentally appropriate and well-functioning equipment and adequate recreational facilities are significant ingredients of milieu treatment.

Phases of Milieu Therapy

Patients who are not prematurely discharged go through several behavioral and treatment phases during the course of hospitalization. Their behavioral vicissitudes within the milieu are theoretically similar to the phases of individual therapy discussed in Chapter 7 and have been outlined by several investigators (Kennedy 1982; Masterson 1972; Rinsley 1980). In short, hospitalization begins with an alliance-building phase, sometimes called the "honeymoon" period, during which all but the most impulsive children control themselves emotionally. When the patient's problems are confronted in therapy and within the milieu, the behavior usually reverts back to that which originally precipitated hospitalization. At that point the second phase, confrontation of the problem, begins. This is a difficult time within the milieu as the patient's grandiose wishes and inappropriate behavior must be understood and effectively managed. As the inpatient process continues and therapy helps patients handle internal conflicts without untoward aggression and acting out, patient behavior within the milieu generally improves. It is usually during this third phase, the internalization phase of milieu therapy, that children are discharged.

Frequently, when the discharge date is set, patients who earlier during treatment had begun to control their problematic behavior seem to lose that control. There is a recycling process in which the recurrence of symptomatic behavior requires the type of limit setting used during the initial part of hospitalization. It is as though patients need reassurance that their previously disruptive behavior will be adequately managed by caregivers outside of the hospital. This interpretation frequently helps to limit this recycling and to focus patients and staff on separation and termination issues.

Termination often leads to resistance not only from the child, but also from the family and the treatment team. Parents worry that they are not prepared for the child's return home and may feel threatened, as the child sometimes does, with the loss of intensive relationships with team members. Team members may complain that the process has moved too quickly and that the child needs more time to internalize gains. Although sometimes valid, it often represents the team's reluctance to discharge a patient whom they know and subsequently admit another patient with whom they will begin the process anew. If the team remains ambivalent about the discharge process, the management of potential patient and family anger related to separation and loss becomes more difficult.

Patient Rights

Although there are variations in due-process procedures for adolescents among different states, children do not have to be judicially committed to psychiatric units when they refuse voluntary admission if their parents or legal guardians agree that hospitalization is necessary. This issue was largely laid to rest by the 1979 Supreme Court decision in *Parham v. J.R.* (1979) that substantiated the previously held presumption that parents will act in the best interests of their children (Appelbaum 1989). However, because of the recent precipitous increase in psychiatric hospitalizations of this age group alluded to in Chapter 4, some commentators have argued that stricter controls are now necessary (Weithorn 1988). Nevertheless, Appelbaum (1989) has suggested that stricter controls are not necessary at this time, noting that the more stringent utilization review criteria currently used by third-party payers may be more effective in limiting inappropriate hospitalizations than would additional legal procedures (see Chapter 15). The adverse effects associated with judicial commitment procedures give credence to Appelbaum's view (Amaya 1991; Amaya and Burlingame 1981).

As noted previously in this chapter, milieu interventions involving the use of seclusion and restraints must follow both Joint Commission on Accreditation of Healthcare Organizations standards and hospital procedures. At the very least, a physician order renewed every 2 to 3 hours (including actual physician supervision), a thorough review of each incident leading to the use of these interventions, a review of how the interventions were applied, and timely consultation with the parents are required. As stated in Chapter 8, prior parental consent for medication usage is necessary except in emergency situations.

All patient rights must be maintained during the course of inpatient treatment. Children have the right to regularly communicate with family members through personal visits, phone contact, and letters. If the team thinks that there are therapeutic reasons to limit the patient's contact with family members, this must be discussed in team meetings and justified in the treatment plan before contact is limited. Of course the patient and family have the right to contest such limitations, either directly with the team or through legal proceedings. If this happens, team members should not feel threatened, but should be willing to participate in a further review to determine what is in the patient's best interest.

Staff-Patient Interactions

The relationships that develop between individual staff members and patients are central to milieu therapy. Just as well-functioning families provide a nurturing holding environment (Winnicott 1975) that strengthens each member's sense of security and capacity for ego growth (instead of the proliferation of primitive defenses), unit workers strive to develop the type of therapeutic community that fosters trust, affective stability, and interpersonal cooperation.

Empathy plays a major role in this process. In order to feel safe and secure, children must know that supervising adults understand their feelings, expressed thoughts, and motives. They turn to special caregivers to determine how good, valuable, and worthy they are. Developmentally appropriate and genuine responses by caregivers positively reflecting child worth enhance self-esteem and substantially contribute to symptom reduction (Baker and Baker 1987). In Chapter 9, the behavioral modification techniques underlying these mirroring responses are discussed.

The physical and emotional availability of staff positively influences the therapeutic process. Unmet patient needs that prior to hospitalization quickly led to anxiety and maladaptive ways of coping are addressed in a timely and appropriate fashion within the unit. This bolsters the nascent sense of trust. Appropriate staff response to patient acting out further enhances the process. Patient behavior must be understood in its clinical context and not taken personally by unit workers, who respond to acting-out behavior in a neutral, nonpunitive, predictable fashion. Staff overreaction only serves to heighten patient misbehavior.

A major unconscious purpose of the inappropriate behaviors seen in children who suffer primarily with interactional problems (i.e., conduct disorder, posttraumatic stress disorder, oppositional disorder, serious pathological character traits) is to continue the cycle of violence, destruction, and humiliation to which most of them have been subjected for years (Dodge et al. 1990). In fact, the reason most of these children are hospitalized is because of the inability of caregivers to interrupt this cycle in less restrictive settings. Within the milieu, unit workers must respond to specific episodes of child destructiveness, violence, or sexual acting out in a different way than the child has come to expect based on previous experience. Instead of responding with anger to anger, or with sexually inappropriate behavior to sexually provocative patient behavior, in a manner that has typically escalated to out-of-control behavior in the patient's experience, unit workers respond appropriately, setting reasonable limits that reestablish security.

Furthermore, child care workers help patients learn how to accept the consequences for their misbehavior. Staff discover how and when to encourage individual patients to comply with milieu interventions. By developing close relationships, staff come to know which patients require "space" as well as how to help particular children manage their punctured narcissism when limits are set and consequences are offered. Although applied predictably, milieu interventions are never applied rigidly. By understanding the differences among children and by striving to help each child master internal, destructive forces through individually designed treatment plans, child care workers promote self-control and emotional growth.

Clinical Staff

Personnel

The American Academy of Child and Adolescent Psychiatry (1990) has outlined the necessary clinical personnel (and their duties) for school-age inpatient units. A child psychiatrist spends at least 5 hours per week in each patient's medical management and treatment, including staff contact, conferences, and therapies. Child psychiatry functions include the admission and discharge of patients, ongoing assessment, supervision of clinical and child care workers, coordination of work with the treatment team, and detailing of patient and family progress in the patient's chart.

At least one social worker for each 10 patients is suggested. Responsibilities include family assessment, social assessment, weekly family-agency contact, participation in discharge planning and treatment team activities, and involvement in family therapy, group therapy, and parent training, as appropriate. The responsibilities of a psychologist include participation in the overall evaluation and treatment process, the implementation of psychological testing as appropriate, and participation in the treatment team. Traditional tasks of the psychologist are changing, however, as psychologists are now admitting their own patients, chairing treatment teams, and sometimes providing the major part of the child's inpatient therapy. Thus, specific tasks depend upon the particular unit and clinical team structure used (see Chapter 15).

At least one psychiatric registered nurse is necessary for 12 patients during active times of the day, while one registered nurse for 50 patients at night meets *minimum* requirements. Nurses participate in daily assessments of the patients, supervision of child care workers, documentation, and the implementation of both the nursing and milieu treatment plans and various therapies, according to unit policy. Child care workers are involved in the behavioral supervision of the patients, maintenance of a safe therapeutic milieu, implementation of specific parts of the treatment plan, and the ongoing assessment and documentation of patient status. Ancillary therapists (activities, music, recreation, occupation, language, art) are important in providing various unit therapies.

Team members perform the clinical duties generally outlined by their respective disciplines and also perform various administrative functions. The duties of the medical director, team leader, and head nurse are examined in Chapter 15.

Staff-Patient Ratio

The number of nursing staff members and child care workers necessary on the unit depends on the unit treatment goals, the variation in patient developmental levels, the length of stay, the acuity and severity of patient symptoms, and the degree of patient impairment. The American Academy of Child and Adolescent Psychiatry (1990) suggests a minimum daytime staff-patient ratio of 1:3 when the main milieu goals are basic observation and maintenance of safety and security. For complex, intensive interventions, a more favorable staff-patient ratio is required. When patients are asleep, a ratio of at least one staff member to six patients is necessary, depending on the number of children within a single living unit and the physical configuration of the unit.

Other investigators report optimal staff-patient ratios of 1:4 during morning activities (Rinsley 1980), 2:5 during mealtimes (Pines et al. 1985), and 4:6 during active, therapeutic programming times (Marsden et al. 1970). Our own experience supports the notion that active milieu therapy requires at least a 1:2 staff-patient ratio.

Communication

Numerous researchers have remarked that the ability of the treatment team to work together as a cohesive body is central to the achievement of the goals and objectives of the milieu therapy program (Feist et al. 1985). In order to provide consistent care hour by hour, day by day, and week by week, staff must work well together. Workers on each shift must know how each patient is responding to the treatment interventions and how the therapies and interventions are subsequently changed in response to patient progress. For example, developmentally disabled patients' behavioral programs may change rapidly as they achieve stated objectives. On one day, staff focus on helping the child hold a spoon, while on the next, after that hurdle is achieved, staff help the patient put food onto the spoon. They then help the patient use the spoon to self-feed (see case example in Chapter 9). Staff members must actively communicate both patient progress and the change in treatment focus. Of course, the same level of communication is necessary when applying milieu interventions in response to patient behavior. This gives the patients a clear message about how misbehavior will be managed and minimizes the possibility of acting out and splitting.

As discussed in Chapter 6, staffings and progress notes promote communication. Nursing meetings and the use of a report book are also very important. On our university unit, the charge nurse writes a paragraph about each patient's behavior during that shift so that all workers during the next shift are aware of changes. The use of the report book fosters continuity throughout the day and has been very successful in enhancing coordination among nursing shifts. Furthermore, nursing meetings at the change of each shift are used to verbally communicate patient progress and to restate treatment objectives and therapeutic and milieu interventions currently in use to promote movement toward those objectives.

Potential Problems

Staff members must be able to tolerate differing views regarding child rearing, rule setting, and the application of consequences. Countertransference feelings, competitive feelings, staff conflict, and lack of training undermine mutual acceptance and respect by staff members and, if not appropriately handled, will subvert the therapeutic process.

Countertransference. Countertransference can be a major problem within the milieu because staff members have their own past experiences that heavily influence how they view patient aggression, oppositionalism, and destructive acting out. Angry, punitive, or overly permissive responses sometimes occur, especially when staff are conflicted about their own past abuse or maltreatment. It is very difficult for some child care workers to empathize with the child's experience of emotional deprivation, physical abuse, and perception of adults as persecutory, reflecting the child's previous failures in social, academic, and interpersonal areas (Berlin et al. 1984; Levinson and Crabtree 1979).

Countertransference can also interfere with the reasonable management of inappropriate, sexualized behaviors. Child care workers and therapists must understand their own underlying sexual issues in order to avoid being vulnerable to patient seductiveness. Underlying discomfort with sexuality often causes staff to respond nontherapeutically. Child care workers sometimes ignore and deny sexual acting out within the milieu. Others become angry and react punitively. Still others tacitly approve of sexual acting out, consciously or unconsciously failing to set reasonable limits.

Countertransference reactions are especially common in response to patient transference itself. The abrupt manner in which some patients shift in their reactions toward staff members from appropriate and kind one minute to hostile and negative the next creates problems for all workers. Patients who use projection and projective identification as an ongoing means of externalizing hostility and provoking those around them to react in a way consonant with their own past experience often elicit negative reactions from staff members.

Competitive feelings. Competitive feelings among staff members that go unnoticed can negatively influence the milieu. These feelings develop between both groups and individuals. An example of the former is illustrated by the sudden disagreements that developed between the day shift and evening shift staff on a unit where we consulted. After the appointment of several new staff members to the evening shift, workers on the two shifts began to increasingly argue and disagree during staffings and milieu meetings as a way of managing anxiety related to their new jobs. Each believed (and stated) that the other shift was either too harsh or too lax. Each strongly projected blame onto the other for the increasing aggression noted on the unit. As always happens during these intrastaff periods of conflict, the patients became aware of the underlying disagreement, which led to disorganization and increased aggression within the milieu. Staff supervision and counseling successfully managed the discord.

Underlying racial tension not recognized or not openly acknowledged can be very destructive. On our state hospital unit we went through a very disruptive period when evening shift child care workers complained that the unit nursing hierarchy had assigned them unnecessarily difficult chores and unfair working schedules because of racial bias. The child care workers were so angry at one point that they impulsively discussed their feelings with a group of patients who subsequently acted out aggressively. Unit security was significantly threatened until the underlying issues were discerned and therapeutically managed.

Negative Patient Reaction to Staff Problems

Patients usually react in negative ways to inappropriate staff behavior. Stanton and Schwartz (1954) used the term "pathological excitement" to describe the increased motor activity, aggressiveness, and mental disorganization seen in patients as a response to staff disagreement (Harper and Geraty 1987). Just as in disturbed families in which children act out unconscious parental wishes and unstated feelings, patients frequently act out staff feelings.

Of course, the most deleterious effect is the disruption of the secure holding environment originally created by positive staff attitude. This seriously limits the unit's ability to provide the necessary elements for a therapeutic community. More than anything else, this inability causes patient insecurity and influences subsequent negative behaviors.

Inappropriate staff behavior during the application of milieu interventions only heightens patient acting out. When staff do not react in a controlled fashion, patients cannot learn to control themselves.

Supervision

Maier and colleagues (1955) recommend a policy of regularly scheduled supervisory conferences for all unit workers that underscores 1) the importance of every aspect of the unit worker's task; 2) the principle that the staff come with a capacity to improve their awareness and skills on the job; 3) the premise that growth is expected regardless of previous training and experience or personal motivation for employment; and 4) the possibility that staff might logically be the key individuals in the treatment of school-age children. Ongoing supervision of all unit workers sends a clear message to everyone that inpatient work with children is very difficult and that even the best-trained workers with the most experience require ongoing assistance and help.

Each child care worker and nursing staff member should be supervised individually at least twice per month, and all unit workers should attend group supervision at least weekly. Unit therapists and senior nursing staff members provide the supervision. Much like the relationship between child care workers and patients, the relationship between the supervisor and milieu staff member is used to build an alliance and to encourage therapeutic interactions during times of reasonable functioning as well as during unit crises.

There are several purposes of supervision. Most important, it provides ongoing training for staff as performance with patients is discussed. Spontaneity and naturalness of interactions are stressed, and unit workers are positively reinforced by supervisors for appropriate nurturing and limit-setting behavior. Interactions between patients and staff, and staff and staff, are closely observed during regular times, as well as during times of crisis. Perceived problems are noted by supervisors and changes are suggested.

Supervision provides an opportunity to explain patient transference to unit staff members. It is important to reframe patient behavior to help child care workers understand that inappropriate behaviors and verbalizations are often transference manifestations and not necessarily personally directed at staff. This reframing helps minimize inappropriate staff counterreactions. For example, one of our female child care workers was having a particularly difficult time with a young male patient who continuously refused to cooperate and led her to feel defeated. She became increasingly frustrated and overreacted to his oppositionalism in ways that only encouraged the escalation of inappropriate behavior. When, through supervision, she realized that the patient's negativism toward her was quite similar to his reactions toward his stepmother, she was able to stop taking the behavior personally and to begin to respond to him therapeutically. This, in turn, helped the patient modify his inappropriate unit behavior.

Supervision is also used to recognize and appropriately manage staff countertransference. Unit staff openly discuss their feelings about both patient behavior and the patients themselves. Staff members are encouraged to explore their own past experiences when necessary to understand feelings about and reactions to patients. The focus of supervision, however, is on the role behaviors and conflicts of the worker, not on personal problems in workers' current, private relationships. If necessary, staff members are referred for their own psychotherapy for such matters.

Supervision is used to handle intrastaff conflict. Unit workers are given the opportunity to discuss issues contributing to discord while supervisors work to understand the underlying issues and to resolve the conflict.

As Scharer and Daverin (1982) have pointed out, supervisors must be aware of their own feelings, attitudes, prejudices, abilities, and limitations. They must be willing to examine their own roles in the supervision process in order to ensure optimal supervision and training.

Of course, child care workers' own past experiences with authority and supervision must be considered by supervisors. The initial phases of supervision often produce defensive reactions on the part of staff members who feel threatened by the process. Supervisors should anticipate this difficulty, giving supervisees the necessary space to process the supervision data.

Choosing Child Care Workers

Obviously, it is very important to choose child care workers carefully, because they are of critical importance to the overall treatment process. Unit administrators must clearly understand what they are looking for in unit workers and must devise a reliable means of determining whether potential candidates meet stated requirements.

Tams' (1982) review of necessary attributes for unit workers is very helpful. Future staff must demonstrate intelligence, the ability to learn, the ability to form deep, meaningful relationships, and the capacity to empathize. They must be able to work in stressful situations, control their impulses, tolerate differences of opinion, and respond to psychologically difficult situations without resorting to primitive defensive maneuvers (i.e., splitting, projection, projective identification, among others).

It is difficult to devise an interview process that adequately and appropriately explores these issues without unduly stressing the interviewee or discouraging the potential unit worker from accepting a position. We encourage a series of interviews with the unit director, head nurse, and one or two unit therapists that explores the candidate's background and particular ways of perceiving life, with special emphasis on past experiences that have influenced development. The candidate's expectations regarding the job and reasons for wanting the position should be explicitly stated. In addition, the individual's self-awareness, self-acceptance, and ability to discuss and describe emotions should all be discerned. How the candidate responds to the interview process, to the interviewer, and to patients and staff members during an initial tour of the unit is also assessed (Tams 1982).

Ideal candidates tend to be males and females in their mid-twenties who are interested in pursuing a career in one of the mental health professions and who see this work as a chance to gain valuable experience. However, we have known many excellent child care workers not represented by these demographics. In our experience, the ideal staff member is someone who likes children, who is psychologically healthy, who can understand what is expected, and who is motivated to perform well.

Staff Training

Initial orientation training and ongoing inservice training are the two principle components of the unit staff development program. Systematic, thorough training is vital to ensure that the therapist, child care workers, and nursing staff members know what is expected and how to implement their tasks and roles.

Orientation training requires multiple sessions over 2 to 3 weeks. Although child care workers are chosen because of their interest and ability to relate to children, training focuses on how to effectively communicate with children, how to listen, how to understand what the child is trying to communicate verbally and nonverbally, and how to respond therapeutically. The orientation sessions specifically review

- The unit philosophy and its underlying psychological principles
- Admission and discharge policies and procedures

- How the milieu program reinforces treatment goals
- The role of the child care worker
- Unit rules and their rationale
- Management of various unit emergencies and precautionary policies
- The use of treatment plans
- The function of particular therapeutic modalities and activities

How and when to apply the various milieu interventions are extensively discussed. A full explanation is given of the point-privilege system and the child care worker's involvement in it. Of course, new staff members learn these procedures both in the classroom and during supervised unit work.

Well-functioning units provide consistent, ongoing training for all staff members. Changes in treatment plans and new therapeutic approaches to be adopted within the unit usually provide ample material and opportunity for inservice training programs. Scharer's (1982) review of inservice topics includes psychopharmacotherapy, cardiopulmonary resuscitation, child psychopathology, psychological development, the use of treatment plans, milieu therapy, dealing with violent patients, active listening, therapeutic holding of the patient, and termination, among others. Bettelheim (1966) emphasizes that ongoing training is necessary for all unit staff, not just child care workers and nursing service members.

Senior staff members, especially the unit director and treatment team leaders, must take every opportunity to model expected behavior and to serve as "teachers" for child care workers and milieu staff members in just the way that child care workers are expected to take every opportunity to interact therapeutically with the patients. Training occurs each time the team leader concisely explains patient and family dynamics in a way that renders the therapeutic components of the treatment plan understandable and logical. It is highly improbable that staff members will actively and positively participate in a treatment plan that does not make sense to them. Staffings should be used to progressively develop an understanding of the patient so that the chosen treatment approaches naturally follow and seem sensible to treatment team members.

Burnout

The insatiable needs of patients, the constant handling of aggression and self-injurious behavior, the intensity of patient explosiveness, the stress implicit in unpredictable patient behavior, the work with angry, rejecting parents, ongoing control issues, staff conflict, periods of understaffing, and frequent changes in personnel all produce the kind of tension and uncertainty that create burnout in unit staff. As Berlin and colleagues (1984) indicate, the hopelessness and helplessness that this stress engenders contribute to staff illness and turnover. Well-developed intrastaff support, sufficient numbers of unit workers, explicit communication, a good inservice training program, effective supervision, and a judicious use of vacation time can serve as preventives or antidotes to these burnout reactions.

References

Aichorn A: Wayward Youth. New York, Viking, 1939

Amaya M: Book review of Child and Adolescent Psychopathology and Involuntary Hospitalization by Crespi T. J Am Acad Child Adolesc Psychiatry 30:160–161, 1991

Amaya M, Burlingame WV: Judicial review of psychiatric admissions: the clinical impact on child and adolescent inpatients. Journal of the American Academy of Child Psychiatry 20:761–776, 1981

American Academy of Child and Adolescent Psychiatry, Task Force on Adolescent Hospitalization: Model for minimum staffing patterns for hospitals providing acute inpatient treatment for children and adolescents with psychiatric illnesses. Washington, DC, American Academy of Child and Adolescent Psychiatry, May 1990

Antoinette T, Iyengar S, Puig-Antich J: Is locked seclusion necessary for children under the age of 14? Am J Psychiatry 147:1283–1289, 1990

Appelbaum PS: Admitting children to psychiatric hospitals: a controversy revived. Hosp Community Psychiatry 40:334–335, 1989

Baker HS, Baker MN: Heinz Kohut's self psychology: an overview. Am J Psychiatry 144:1–9, 1987

Berlin I, Critchley D, Rossman P: Current concepts in milieu treatment of seriously disturbed children and adolescents. Psychotherapy 21:118–131, 1984

Bettelheim B: Training the child-care worker in a residential center. Am J Orthopsychiatry 36:694–705, 1966

Bettelheim B, Sylvester E: Milieu therapy: indications and illustrations. Psychoanalytic Review 36:54–68, 1949

Binder RI: The use of seclusion on an inpatient crisis intervention unit. Hosp Community Psychiatry 30:266–269, 1979

Dalton R, Muller B, Forman M: The psychiatric hospitalization of children: an overview. Child Psychiatry Hum Dev 19:231–244, 1989

Dodge K, Bates J, Pettit G: Mechanisms in the cycle of violence. Science 250:1678–1683, 1990

Erickson W, Realmuto G: The frequency of seclusion in an adolescent psychiatric unit. J Clin Psychol 44:238–241, 1983

Feist J, Slowiak C, Colligan R: Beyond good intentions: applying scientific methods to the art of milieu therapy. Residential Group Care and Treatment 3:13–32, 1985

Gallagher M, Mittelstadt P, Slater B: Establishing time-out procedures in a day treatment facility for young children. Residential Treatment for Children and Youth 5:59–68, 1988

Garrison WT, Ecker B, Friedman M, et al: Aggression and counteraggression during child psychiatric hospitalization. J Am Acad Child Adolesc Psychiatry 29:242–250, 1990

Gerlock A, Solomons H: Factors associated with the seclusion of psychiatric patients. Perspect Psychiatr Care 21:47–53, 1983

Gutheil TG: Observations on the theoretical bases for seclusion of the psychiatric inpatient. Am J Psychiatry 135:325–328, 1978

Harper G, Geraty R: Hospital and residential treatment (ch 64), in Psychiatry, Vol 2. Edited by Michels R, Cooper AM, Guze SB, et al. Philadelphia, PA, JB Lippincott, 1987

Irwin M: Literature review, in Psychiatric Hospitalization of Children. Edited by Schulman JL, Irwin M. Springfield, IL, Charles C Thomas, 1982, pp 5–42

Jones R, Downing R, Miller P, et al: Time-out normative data: frequency and duration with child psychiatry inpatients. Poster session at the annual meeting of the American Academy of Child and Adolescent Psychiatry, Chicago, IL, October 1990

Joshi PT, Capozzoli JA, Coyle JT: Use of a quiet room on an inpatient unit. J Am Acad Child Adolesc Psychiatry 27:642–644, 1988

Kennedy PA: Phases of milieu therapy, in Psychiatric Hospitalization of Children. Edited by Schulman JL, Irwin M. Springfield, IL, Charles C Thomas, 1982, pp 119–128

Levinson DF, Crabtree LH Jr: Ward tension and staff leadership in a therapeutic community for hospitalized adolescents. Psychiatry 42:220–240, 1979

Maier HW, Hilgeman LM, Shugart G, et al: The role of residential treatment for children, 7: supervision of child care workers in a residential treatment service. Am J Orthopsychiatry 25:699–704, 1955

Marsden G, McDermott JF, Miner D: Residential treatment of children: a survey of institutional characteristics. Journal of the American Academy of Child Psychiatry 9:332–346, 1970

Masterson J: Treatment of the Borderline Adolescent: A Developmental Approach. New York, Wiley, 1972

Millstein KH, Cotton NS: Predictors of the use of seclusion on an inpatient child psychiatric unit. J Am Acad Child Adolesc Psychiatry 29:256–264, 1990

Parham v JR, 442 U.S. 584 (1979)

Parmelee D: The adolescent and the young adult, in Inpatient Psychiatry: Diagnosis and Treatment, 2nd Edition. Edited by Sederer LI. Baltimore, MD, Williams & Wilkins, 1986, pp 280–295

Phillips P, Nasr SJ: Seclusion and restraint and prediction of violence. Am J Psychiatry 140:229–232, 1983

Pines R, Kupst M, Natta M, et al: Staff-patient ratio and type of interaction on a child psychiatry inpatient unit. Child Psychiatry Hum Dev 16:14–29, 1985

Redl F: The concept of a "therapeutic milieu." Am J Orthopsychiatry 29:721–736, 1959

Rinsley DB: Theory and practice of intensive residential treatment of adolescents (Fifth Annual Edward A Strecker Memorial Lecture, October 14, 1968), in Adolescent Psychiatry, Vol 1: Development and Clinical Studies. Edited by Feinstein SC, Giovacchini PL, Miller AA. New York, Basic Books, 1971, pp 479–509

Rinsley D: Principles of therapeutic milieu with children, in Treatment of Emotional Disorders in Children and Adolescents. Edited by Sholevar G, Benson R, Blinder B. New York, SP Medical and Scientific Books, 1980, pp 191–208

Scharer K: In-service training, in Psychiatric Hospitalization of Children. Edited by Schulman JL, Irwin M. Springfield, IL, Charles C Thomas, 1982, pp 335–338

Scharer K, Daverin AG: Staff supervision, in Psychiatric Hospitalization of Children. Edited by Schulman JL, Irwin M. Springfield, IL, Charles C Thomas, 1982, pp 339–349

Soloff PH, Turner S: Patterns of seclusion: a prospective study. J Nerv Ment Dis 169:37–44, 1981

Stanton A, Schwartz M: The Mental Hospital. New York, Basic Books, 1954

Stone LA: Residential treatment, in Basic Handbook of Child Psychiatry, Vol 3: Therapeutic Interventions. Edited by Harrison SI (JD Noshpitz, Editor-in-Chief). New York, Basic Books, 1979, pp 231–262

Tams PA: The staff, in Psychiatric Hospitalization of Children. Edited by Schulman JL, Irwin M. Springfield, IL, Charles C Thomas, 1982, pp 54–62

Weithorn L: Mental hospitalization of troublesome youth: an analysis of skyrocketing admission rates. Stanford Law Review 40:773–838, 1988

Wherry J: The therapeutic use of seclusion with children and adolescents. Residential Treatment for Children and Youth 4:51–61, 1986

Wilson M, Soth N: Testing milieu principles and treatment philosophy. Residential Treatment for Children and Youth 4:21–24, 1986

Winnicott D: The depressive position in normal emotional development, in Collected Papers: Through Paediatrics to Psycho-Analysis. London, Hogarth Press, 1975, pp 262–277

Chapter 13

Special Clinical and Developmental Issues

In this chapter we discuss clinical problems and age-related considerations that must be specifically addressed on school-age units. We do not review all aspects of these issues, but selectively describe the pertinent diagnostic, milieu, and treatment components.

Aggression

Aggressive behavior, including physical assault, self-injury, property damage, verbal hostility, and noncompliance, is seen in over 70% of our university unit patients and in over 80% of our state hospital patients. Anticipation represents the first step for managing inpatient aggression. Recent studies have addressed patient, family, staff, and environment characteristics that are predictive of inpatient aggression (Garrison 1984). Gender, age, and psychological status have all been shown to be important. Boys are more assaultive than girls (Pfeffer et al. 1983), although girls self-injure more often (Garrison et al. 1990). Recent and past aggression, as well as recent and past psychopathology, are also predictors, especially in younger children, as are poor impulse control, poor reality testing, the concept of death as temporary, the use of projection as a defense mechanism (Pfeffer et al. 1987), paranoid thinking, and the presence of neurological signs and symptoms (Lewis et al. 1984). Furthermore, the likelihood of violence is increased when two or more of the variables coexist (Pfeffer et al. 1987). Family factors have also been shown to be predictive by Lewis and colleagues (1984), who found an association between childhood inpatient violence and parental aggression.

Garrison and colleagues (1990) have noted that various settings affect aggression. They report that transitions occurring during the hospital day as well as less structured activities and locations are associated with unit aggression. Violence was less likely during the first 5 days of hospitalization. In our experience, staff-patient ratio, staff attitude (especially when managing unit aggression), inappropriate milieu controls, and negative group behavior can all promote the development of inpatient aggression. The Child Behavior Checklist (CBCL) (Achenbach and Edelbrock 1983) aggression subscale is a useful predictor of inpatient violence and destruction (see Chapter 6). It facilitates the early identification of potentially aggressive patients so that treatment plans can be formulated accordingly.

Out-of-control aggression can be very destructive within the milieu and can engender feelings of insecurity in other patients. Impulse-ridden patients are then more likely to become aggressive and difficult to manage. Anxious children become frightened. Needy, dependent children mimic aggression, especially self-injurious behavior, when they see how much attention these behaviors elicit. If unit violence and self-destruction are chronic and persistent, the milieu, in and of itself, becomes countertherapeutic and directly damaging to patients.

Particular incidents of aggressive behavior should be managed therapeutically by using accepted behavioral modification techniques and principles (see Chapter 9), by enforcing consequences, by rewarding incompatible, desirable alternatives, and by ignoring some kinds of minor behaviors that are not blatantly dangerous or destructive (Werry and Wollersheim 1989). Positive reinforcement for nonaggressive behavior should be stressed, but very clear limits must be set at the time of the aggressive behavior for adequate control. Furthermore, the staff must teach patients alternative ways of expressing anger and underlying rage (see Chapter 12).

Although recent studies indicate that counteraggressive milieu interventions do not significantly alter long-term acting-out behavior (Garrison et al. 1990), it is nevertheless important that staff react quickly to aggressive incidents, reestablishing order and reassuring other patients. The specific intervention by staff depends on the type of aggression expressed, its potential dangers, and unit policy and procedures (see Chapter 12). Understanding the association between patient aggression and particular symptom and diagnostic clusters is necessary to plan effective milieu responses.

Anxiety

About 10% of inpatients have an anxiety disorder (Alessi and Magen 1988). However, anxious children rarely act out aggressively. When they do, it is usually a response to sudden, panicky feelings associated with separation anxiety or agitation seen in posttraumatic stress disorder. The behavior is managed by verbal intervention and possibly by removing the patient from the situation. The use of more restrictive interventions is not necessary. Benzodiazepines, especially alprazolam, are useful for both acute and ongoing treatment.

Oppositionalism

Most inpatients violate everyday rules and present with provocative behavior and stubbornness at some point during their hospitalization. Intermittent noncompliance can represent underlying frustration in a child who has not learned more appropriate ways of expressing distress, although chronic oppositionalism is almost always a sign of underlying psychopathology. These children are passively resistant and verbally aggressive, though nonviolent and usually nondestructive. They thrive on interpersonal conflict and often know exactly what to say to annoy or anger others. Within the milieu, their oppositional behavior should initially be ignored. If it becomes persistent, verbal correction and removal of the patient from the situation are appropriate. Time out is administered for flagrant violations of the rules, and isolation is used when these violations persist. More restrictive interventions and the use of medications are unnecessary.

Conduct Disorder

Patients with conduct disorder become aggressive during times of intrapsychic and interpersonal conflict. Because they typically act out underlying fears and concerns in nonverbal ways, the cause of each destructive and violent act must be considered in order to determine what the patient is trying to communicate. In fact, a major purpose for the hospitalization of these children is to clarify what they are struggling to express.

Children with the solitary subtype of conduct disorder present with unsocialized behavior, frequently act in hostile ways toward others, and are impulsively aggressive when among other children. They may demonstrate out-of-control behavior when stressed. On the other hand, children in the group subtype are more sociable but are verbally hostile and frequently try to intimidate vulnerable patients. They may physically resist unit authority and are especially susceptible to acting out intrastaff conflict. Inadequate unit supervision often leads these patients to act destructively and violently in groups.

Aggressive behaviors should not be ignored within the milieu. Verbal correction and removal of the patient are used at times of interpersonal disagreement and when staff anticipate escalating conflict. Time out is administered for discrete acts of aggression that are not part of an ongoing pattern of misbehavior. Isolation is used to manage repeated verbal threats directed toward other patients and staff. Recidivistic flare-ups of violence or destruction are managed with seclusion. Locked seclusion is chosen for nonpsychotic patients who refuse unlocked seclusion. Full (five-way) restraints are used for out-of-control violence that cannot otherwise be managed (see Chapter 12).

In periods of acute agitation, benzodiazepines are appropriately used to help reduce patient agitation. Neuroleptics should be reserved for use when a central ego disintegrative defect is noted. Of course, the presence of such a defect as inferred by patient delusions and hallucinations means that the aggressive behavior is due to an underlying psychotic disorder, not conduct disorder.

Depression

Depressed patients become agitated and short-tempered, but rarely violent toward others. During periods of extreme agitation, they sometimes impulsively attempt to hurt themselves. Ignoring this behavior within the milieu is always inappropriate. Cognitive-behavioral verbal correction is necessary, as is removal from the situation because of agitation. Physical intervention at times of self-abuse should be timely and effective. Isolation, seclusion, and the use of restraints are contraindicated with depressed children. The pharmacotherapeutic management of nonpsychotic acutely depressed children is reviewed in Chapter 8.

Mania

Manic children may react aggressively when limits are set on grandiose wishes. Child care workers and therapists often can anticipate such episodes as they observe escalating hypomanic behavior. Verbal correction and removal of the patient from the situation are the first steps to modify inappropriate behavior. Time out is inappropriate with manic aggression because the underlying pressure to act out is beyond the control of the child, who will not stay in time out. With increasing agitation leading to actual aggression, manic patients should be placed in unlocked seclusion with a child care worker. Full restraints are used for out-of-control violence that does not respond to less restrictive measures.

The combination of lithium carbonate and a neuroleptic medication is often necessary for manic patients who act out violently and destructively. Although the combination of lithium carbonate and carbamazepine has been shown to be effective with rapidly cycling, aggressive manic adults, we have not found this combination to be helpful with children, and there is an anecdotal report in the literature that this combination can actually contribute to increased aggression (Myers and Carrera 1989).

Borderline Personality Traits

Children with borderline personality traits often try to engage staff members in verbal sparring. Like conduct-disordered children, they react with impulsive aggression to unit authority. Unlike conduct-disordered children, however, their aggression escalates to the point of self-abuse. When consequences are enforced for violations of rules within the milieu, borderline patients may react by hurting themselves and thus sabotaging the milieu intervention plan.

Within the milieu, a certain amount of nonviolent, nondestructive borderline behavior must be ignored. Verbal correction and removal from the situation are used for persistent verbal sparring. When these patients violate major unit rules in a nonviolent manner, time out is implemented. Repeated violations that have not responded to the therapeutic implementation of time out should lead to isolation of the patient. Seclusion and restraints should be avoided, if possible, as they appear to provoke self-injurious behavior in these patients. Very clear, specific consequences must be set for borderline patients with self-injurious behavior. This behavior should be immediately interrupted by staff, who physically hold the patient until calm. Milieu interventions are designed to contain these patients until the development of a therapeutic alliance and progress in psychodynamic therapy can help reduce the pressures contributing to the self-injurious behavior. Psychopharmacotherapy is usually ineffective, except when these patients present with psychotic episodes. In those times, the judicious use of neuroleptics can be helpful in reestablishing effective reality testing.

Organic Personality Syndrome, Organic Mood Syndrome, and Pervasive Developmental Disorder

Patients with organic personality syndrome, organic mood syndrome, and pervasive developmental disorder often present with a range of serious, self-directed aggression including eye gouging, head banging, self-hitting, and ingestion of inappropriate objects, among others. Aggression toward others is usually limited to impulsive hitting and kicking, although some organically impaired patients repeatedly victimize the same individual.

Self-injurious behavior should never be ignored. However, after chronic exposure to self-injurious behavior, staff tend to overlook repeated episodes of self-directed aggression. Supervision becomes lax, leaving these patients more vulnerable to additional episodes of self-injurious behavior. When these patients are agitated, they should be removed from the situation. Single incidents of outwardly directed aggression should be managed via well supervised time out; however, this intervention should not be used for self-injurious behavior. Repeated aggression and all episodes of self-injurious behavior should lead to well-supervised isolation (see Chapter 12). During that time a child care worker who has a working alliance with the patient monitors the situation closely and physically intervenes when the patient self-abuses. Seclusion without the presence of a child care worker is inappropriate because these patients will increase their self-stimulatory, self-abusive behaviors while alone. Waist restraints can be used as part of a proactively created treatment plan for continual self-injurious behavior. These patients must be continually visually monitored, however, for their ongoing protection.

Farber's (1987) recent review of the pharmacotherapy of self-injurious behavior in mentally retarded patients nicely summarizes current approaches. Wysocki (1984) advances realistic caveats about the drug treatment of self-injurious behavior. The clinician must consider the possibility of side effects, the suppression of positive behaviors as well as negative ones, the possibility of overlooking environmental causes of the self-injurious behavior, the lack of knowledge about the neurochemistry of self-injurious behavior, and the absence of studies underscoring the efficacy of pharmacotherapy with patients exhibiting self-injurious behavior (Farber 1987).

Psychosis

Psychotic patients sometimes present with unpredictable aggression. At other times, they react to stress with out-of-control behavior involving both outwardly directed aggression and self-abuse. This behavior should not be ignored within the milieu. Verbal correction and removal with the provision of one-to-one staff attention are necessary for all actively psychotic children. Child care workers must function as auxiliary egos and facilitators for these patients and must be sensitive to individual differences among psychotic patients in capacity, motivation, and level of communication (Cantor and Kestenbaum 1986). Especially disruptive psychotic patients should be isolated in their own rooms with child care worker supervision to guard against patient injury and to foster the establishment of an alliance. Seclusion is inappropriate unless the patient becomes destructive, at which time supervised seclusion may be necessary. Full restraints are only used during out-of-control, aggressive episodes when less restrictive measures and pharmacotherapeutic approaches are unsuccessful. Drug management with neuroleptics is a central focus of treatment (see Chapter 12). The addition of a benzodiazepine is often helpful with acute, psychotic agitation.

Multiple Diagnoses

There are also specific combinations of diagnoses that are frequently associated with inpatient aggression. Conduct disorder and depression, post-traumatic stress disorder and conduct disorder, affective disorder with psychosis, and organic personality syndrome and conduct disorder are four combinations that often have a potentiating effect on both violent and destructive acting out. The occurrence of dual diagnoses must be considered in each case so that subsequent treatment plans can be developed accordingly, as in the following case example:

> Bobby H., 10 years of age, was referred for hospitalization when his destructive behavior, including aggression against his younger siblings and mother, could not be contained in outpatient therapy. Although he was said to have always had a difficult temperament, he became openly oppositional during first grade. He subsequently developed increasingly violent behavior following the death of his paternal grandfather a year prior to admission. His symptoms escalated from that point until admission. The evaluation revealed that Bobby's behavior resulted from conduct disorder, dysthymic disorder, and pathological character traits. Bobby's parents were extremely punitive, but also impulsive and inconsistent in their attempts to deal with his aggression.
>
> The patient was admitted for the purpose of disrupting this escalating cycle of destructive and violent behavior, and to teach his parents to recognize the precipitants of the aggression and to develop different, more appropriate responses to them. A treatment plan was designed to therapeutically manage those behaviors and to treat underlying psychopathological disorders in family members contributing to the presenting problems.
>
> Within the milieu, our initial strategy involved the development of an alliance with Bobby by two primary caregivers. Unit rules were clearly explained and positive inducements and reinforcers for appropriate behavior outlined. A hierarchy of interventions was devised by team members, including verbal intervention by staff during times of peer conflict and arguments, separation from others when agitated and verbally aggressive, and the use of time out for physical aggression. Child care workers were instructed to hold Bobby in the manner explained in Chapter 12 if he refused to comply. Of course, the milieu and unit therapy approaches typically used for other children were also used for Bobby and his family.
>
> Bobby responded fairly well to the techniques employed to manage his aggression. On three occasions during the second and third weeks following admission, he required holding by staff members (once for an hour) until he would comply with time-out procedures. After a hospitalization of 56 days,

and with good participation by his family in the treatment plan, he was able to return home and to school without a major recurrence of the type of aggression that had originally precipitated hospitalization.

Other Disruptive Behaviors

Stealing, lying, runaway behavior, fire setting, and truancy are often seen in behaviorally disordered patients. Stealing and lying, though frequent, are not primary reasons for admission, in and of themselves. Theft often has both psychological and sociological antecedents, but should be successfully inhibited in a well-designed milieu. The same is true for truancy.

Fire Setting

The prevalence of fire setting in children who are subsequently hospitalized is 12%–14% (Dalton et al. 1986; Stewart and Culver 1982). Nevertheless, fire setting is rarely the main reason for hospitalization. Families, especially disorganized ones, often struggle to maintain the fire-setter within the home through vigilance and by trying to minimize the symptom.

School-age fire-setters usually act alone, often setting fires in their bedroom or in a closet at home. Through the years, theorists have offered a variety of explanations for this clinical phenomenon. Currently, emphasis is placed on conflict over aggression and curiosity, two prominent variables contributing to this symptom (Fineman 1980; Kolko and Kazdin 1991). For many of these children, fire setting represents a psychological compromise used to externalize aggressive feelings in chaotic families who, on the surface, appear to be nurturing, but who are not really able to meet the child's needs. In adolescents, this symptom is usually a delinquent behavior, in response to a desire for revenge, and is often carried out within a group. Fire setting in both age groups typically accompanies a diagnosis of conduct disorder.

Within the milieu, staff must make sure that matches and cigarette lighters are kept out of the way. This symptom, however, usually responds very quickly to removal of the child from the home. In fact, during the past 5 years, there have been no reported incidents of fire setting on either our university or our state hospital units. Many fire-setters behave very passively within the milieu. They are unable to understand their own wishes or to verbally express their needs. Some readily play fireman and seem obsessed with the theme, whereas others do not spontaneously mention fire and shy away from a discussion when asked.

In addition to securing the milieu, treatment includes family therapy, individual therapy, assertiveness training, and liaison work within the community. The top inpatient priority is to establish an alliance with the patient through which feelings can be explored and understood. Family therapy is crucial. Understanding the source of the family disorganization is necessary to determine whether the patient will be able to immediately return home following discharge. Assertiveness training and various social skills approaches are also necessary to help the patient understand underlying feelings that are acted out via this symptom and to develop new, healthier ways of expression. Finally, involvement of local fire officials to explain the do's and don't's regarding fire within the community can be very helpful.

Although good efficacy studies are not available, it is our experience that about one-fourth of these patients do not give up this symptom, but instead become recalcitrant fire-setters. About half of our fire-setters have been referred to out-of-home, less restrictive settings following hospitalization because of ongoing family instability (Dalton et al. 1986).

Runaway Behavior

Children run away both from home and from inpatient units. There are two primary reasons for running away from home. The first is to escape abuse and aggression. The second reflects psychopathology in the child and is almost always a sign of very disturbed object relations. Children who try to run away from inpatient units are usually either expressing their underlying or overt conflict with authority or trying to assuage feelings secondary to separation anxiety.

Often, one-to-one staff attention is necessary to adequately maintain these children. When patients threaten to escape or when their behavior suggests that they will run away if given a chance, they should be restricted to the unit until appropriate alliance building in both individual psychotherapy and within the milieu can be used to establish a contract with the patient and, subsequently, to understand and treat the underlying issues. Runaway precautions, like suicide precautions (see below), should be removed cautiously, only after staff feel more secure about the patient's active involvement in the milieu program. Seclusion and restraints are inappropriate interventions for managing this symptom.

Sexual Abuse and Sexual Acting Out

Recent studies have indicated that 16% of boys and 48% of girls admitted to child psychiatry inpatient units have been sexually abused (Kohan et al.

1987). The abuse includes intercourse, oral-genital contact, digital penetration, and involvement in pornography. Characteristic behaviors of sexually abused children that are seen during hospitalization include sex play with others, seductiveness with staff members, sexualized talk, masturbation, verbalization of hurtful and violent thoughts, and violent behavior, as well as withdrawn and suicidal behavior. Symptoms of posttraumatic stress disorder (PTSD), including a reexperiencing of the abuse, avoidance behaviors, and autonomic hyperarousal, are also frequently seen. McLeer and colleagues (1988) found that 48% of sexually abused inpatients met DSM-III-R (American Psychiatric Association 1987) criteria for PTSD. Seventy-five percent of the children who were abused by natural fathers, 67% of those abused by strangers, 25% of those abused by trusted adults, but none who were abused by other children, met the PTSD criteria. Associated diagnoses included developing personality problems, conduct disorder, oppositional disorder, and mood disorder. The Child Behavior Checklist (CBCL) is quite useful in elucidating PTSD, while the Children's Depression Inventory (CDI) (Kovacs 1980), the State-Trait Anxiety Inventory for Children (STAIC) (Spielberger 1973), and the CBCL as well, help identify sexually abused children with other diagnoses (McLeer et al. 1988).

Emergency rooms in children's hospitals frequently admit cases of suspected sexual abuse to their pediatric or psychiatric units. It is then incumbent on the treatment team to fully evaluate the possible occurrence of abuse and its effects. During the past 3 years we have evaluated three children for suspected sexual abuse on our university unit, although we have treated many more who were hospitalized after their sexual abuse had already been discovered.

Guidelines proposed by the American Academy of Child and Adolescent Psychiatry (1988) are very helpful when evaluating children who are known or suspected to have been sexually abused. In short, the child should be seen for the minimum number of evaluation sessions and by the fewest number of people necessary to determine whether abuse has occurred. Interviewing and gathering a history from both parents are very important. In custody disputes, a guardian ad litem should be appointed to represent the child's best interests. The possibility of false allegations should always be considered. A clinician should observe the child separately with each parent, after meeting initially with the child to establish an alliance and to impart to the child a sense of control. Of course, the child's credibility should be assessed. Factors enhancing credibility include detailed descriptions in the child's own language and from the child's point of view, spontaneity, an appropriate degree of anxiety, consistency of the allegations over time, behavioral changes consistent with the abuse, and an absence of motivation or undue influence for fabrication. The use of anatomical dolls is not necessary but can be useful for eliciting the child's terminology for anatomical parts. Coaching or instructing the child with the dolls is specifically contraindicated. Spontaneous drawings may be quite useful and revealing. Videotaping is sometimes helpful to avoid duplication of efforts and to preserve the child's initial statements. A physical examination is always indicated when sexual abuse is suspected.

Seductive behaviors as well as direct sexual acting out can be very disruptive within the milieu and often create major countertransference problems (see Chapter 12). Sexualized behaviors provoke out-of-control behaviors in other children. Staff must immediately set appropriate limits. Child care workers should remove children behaving in a sexually inappropriate manner and clearly describe which behaviors are inappropriate and why they are inappropriate. Staff must avoid guilt- and shame-inducing statements and feelings. Previously defined consequences are enforced. Often one-to-one supervision is necessary for children compelled to act out sexually. There must be an adequate number of well-trained and well-supervised staff members to control this behavior, especially on large units where a number of children share dormitory-like rooms.

The goals for hospitalization of the sexually abused child include a full understanding of subsequent behavioral and psychological sequelae, the development of a therapeutic alliance, and the remission of the most pernicious behaviors and symptoms precipitating hospitalization. The family's capacity to protect the child must also be assessed, and if defective, an alternative posthospital placement must be obtained through child protective services. Behavioral, family, and individual psychotherapies must be creatively combined to adequately treat these patients. The cognitive-behavioral treatment approach described by Deblinger and colleagues (1990) (see Chapter 9) is an example of currently used behavioral treatment. Family work always includes appropriate parent training designed to help family members recognize and therapeutically respond to PTSD, other disorders, and sexual acting-out symptoms within the home. Individual psychotherapy designed to build an alliance and to confront internal fears and externalizing behaviors is often necessary with those children who have incorporated the traumatic abuse into their developing personality structure. Therapists must understand how compulsive sexual acting out is both a defense against previous trauma and a misguided expression of the need for nurturance. This is gently interpreted in response to sexualized behaviors during therapy sessions.

Public displays of masturbation are frequently seen on school-age units by both sexually abused and nonsexually abused children. Younger, developmentally needy children sometimes rub their genitals in a self-soothing way much as other children suck their thumbs. Sexually abused boys and girls sometimes masturbate as a way of communicating the wish to sexually act out or as a way of unconsciously communicating anxiety. Unsocialized children often present with this behavior because they have not learned appropriate social limits. Older children use masturbation on occasion as a way of violating unit rules. Although the behavior must be understood according to each patient's needs, it is advisable that child care workers clearly explain that public masturbation is not acceptable social behavior and that masturbation should be confined to periods when the child is alone.

Suicidal Ideation and Behavior

About 40% of our patients during the past 5 years have threatened to hurt or kill themselves either prior to hospitalization or during their inpatient stay. Six percent actually made bona fide attempts prior to admission. Three of our last 300 inpatients have seriously tried to hurt themselves in the hospital while verbalizing suicidal wishes: one tried to strangle himself and two others engaged in severe head banging, all while saying they wanted to kill themselves.

Numerous psychological, family, and environmental variables have been associated with both suicidal ideation and actual suicidal behavior. Factors influencing suicidal ideation include depression, preoccupation with death, and general psychopathology. These variables and others are related to actual suicidal behavior in school-age children. Older white males (11- to 12-year-olds) are more likely to attempt suicide than younger children (Brent and Kolko 1990). Family characteristics such as lack of generational boundaries, marital discord, symbiotic parent-child relationships, and high family conflict with low family achievement are correlated with suicidal behavior (Campbell 1990). Sexual abuse, exposure to suicidal behavior, early losses and stresses, and epilepsy are also contributants (Cohen-Sandler et al. 1982).

The cultural myth that children do not kill themselves has followed the generally accepted view that preadolescents do not understand the irreversible nature of suicide. Recent studies have shown that school-age children, in general, are surprisingly knowledgeable about the subject. The major difference between children and adolescents lies in the congruence among knowledge, fantasy, and method. Adolescents know what acts will lead to death and the necessary ingredients to commit those acts, as well as what will likely happen if they actually do commit one of those acts. Prepubertal children, on the other hand, have shown discrepancies between what they know to be a suicidal act and their fantasies of what will kill and what will not (Carlson et al. 1987). Among nonhospitalized preadolescents, jumping from heights is the most frequent means of suicide, followed by self-poisoning, hanging, stabbing, and running into traffic. There is no currently available information about the methods used by patients while hospitalized.

Two principal steps are necessary for managing suicidal behavior within the milieu. First, a thorough clinical evaluation must be carried out, supplemented by the use of the Diagnostic Interview Schedule for Children (DISC) and the Spectrum of Suicidal Behavior (SSB) Scale (Campbell 1990; Pfeffer 1986). The level of hopelessness and helplessness as well as the possibility of depression, psychosis, bipolar illness, substance abuse, and paranoid ideation must be closely examined. The patient's ongoing suicidal ideation must be continuously assessed. If the suicidal threat continues, the therapist must discern whether the patient has a plan; if so, its lethality should be determined. An assessment of the family members is necessary, including their original contributions to the patient's suicidal behavior as well as their current views of the behavior. Second, the patient must be continually observed within the milieu during each shift until suicidal behavior is no longer a threat. Removal of visual contact should be gradual. The treatment team must anticipate times and activities that might facilitate suicidal behavior and react accordingly. The following case is illustrative:

> Jake, a 12-year-old, was admitted to the unit with an extensive personal history of dysphoric behavior and a family history of depression. He was diagnosed as suffering with major depression, precipitated by the death of his grandfather. His parents sought hospitalization after Jake expressed the wish to die "to be with [his] grandfather again." He told his mother that he planned to jump from the roof of their home.
>
> Despite the treatment team's vigilance regarding his suicide potential, Jake tried to strangle himself while showering during his third hospital day. He had earlier hidden a coat hanger behind the toilet in the bathroom. Although Jake was supposed to be continually supervised, the child care worker had stepped out of the bathroom to attend to two other children who were arguing. When the worker returned 1 minute later, Jake was discovered wrapping the coat hanger around his neck. He was removed, unhurt, from the shower.
>
> The following morning the treatment team met and reaffirmed Jake's ongoing need for continual visual contact, which was to include bathroom time and time asleep, as well as the remainder of Jake's day. Individual psychotherapy, pharmacotherapy, activities therapy, group cognitive-behavioral therapy, and family therapy were included in his treatment plan and then implemented.
>
> After 2 weeks, the patient's affect brightened as his depression abated. Our evaluation at that time revealed that Jake did not actively think about killing himself the way he had at the time of admission. He readily agreed to a no-suicide contract (Brent and Kolko 1990). Also, his family had been actively engaged in the treatment process. He asked that he be allowed to join

in off-unit activities. This was allowed on a limited basis, with ongoing continual supervision, only after his therapist and the treatment team concluded that Jake's feelings of hopelessness and helplessness had begun to remit and that he was no longer actively suicidal.

After another week, when there had been no incidents, Jake was allowed to play with the other children in the unit day room without continual visual contact. During this time, however, he was required to make contact with the unit charge nurse every 5 minutes. The time increment was increased by 5 minutes each three days until Jake was allowed to play with the other children for 30 consecutive minutes without direct, active staff contact. At that point, after an alliance had been formed and Jake's affect had significantly improved (5 weeks following admission), he was taken off of suicide precautions.

Encopresis

Encopresis is the passage of feces into inappropriate places at any age after bowel control is usually established. This predominantly male disorder affects approximately 1% of 5-year-olds. Chronic soiling may persist from infancy onward (primary), or it may appear as a regressive phenomenon (secondary). It is often associated with chronic constipation, fecal impaction, and overflow incontinence, and may progress to psychogenic megacolon. Twenty of our last 300 patients, all male, have presented with encopretic symptoms during hospitalization.

Nonorganic encopresis is associated with various behavioral and characterological problems. Encopresis is often related to unresolved separation-individuation issues that patients ineffectively try to manage in a psychologically controlling fashion. This, paradoxically, contributes to frequent out-of-control behavior, of which encopresis is only one example. Some encopretic patients present with obstinate but nonassertive behaviors and are unable to verbally express and understand their own feelings. They act out both impulsively and aggressively. Others present with passive-aggressive behavior, appear to be developmentally regressed and behaviorally disorganized though not psychotic, and come from very disorganized and abusive families. All patients deny their encopretic symptoms, frequently trying to hide soiled underwear and feces. Their insistent denial is an attempt to avoid feelings of shame, which is a pervasive affect related to their struggles for autonomy and control (Erikson 1963).

Within the milieu, just as within the community, children with encopresis are often derided by peers. Their associated behavioral and personality problems also contribute to difficult peer relationships. Staff frustration with messiness and underlying patient anger lead to countertransference problems. Child care workers sometimes resent having to check these patients' hygiene habits so closely. Both staff and peers have difficulty with the projected rage typical of encopretic patients.

Specific milieu treatment approaches for secondary encopresis include the use of mineral oil and a high-fiber diet. The patient sits on the toilet for 10 to 15 minutes following each meal and is rewarded specifically for sitting on the toilet, for good behavior during the process, and for a bowel movement. The child and unit primary caregiver record patient progress.

The treatment of primary encopresis is somewhat different. Often the colon must initially be evacuated via the use of enemas. A program is then established in which the child sits on the toilet each morning and is given a reward for a bowel movement. If the patient does not produce a reasonable amount (one half cup), a glycerine suppository is inserted. The patient then has breakfast and, following a short period of time, returns to sit on the toilet. The patient is rewarded for success. If unsuccessful, the patient is given an enema but is not rewarded. However, no more than two enemas per week are used. The child's clothes are examined at the end of the day. If not soiled, an additional reward is given. If soiled, the patient receives a predetermined consequence. The main difficulty with this plan lies in finding suitable rewards to enhance the development of self-toileting skills. This approach requires both patience and consistency.

For those patients who only show fecal streaking in their underwear, a psychoeducational approach is used initially, with staff observing the child's postelimination hygiene and retraining the patient when necessary. Patients who initially present with diarrhea-like stools because of a partial impaction will require a mild, consistently used laxative. A pediatric gastroenterology consultation is indicated for the treatment of megacolon and fecal impaction, and when underlying organic pathology is suspected.

Unit workers must have clear expectations of the encopretic child. Disorganized patients are taught assertiveness skills in both the milieu and group therapies. Child care workers try to maintain an effective balance between limit setting and negotiation with obstinate patients. Positive reinforcements are very important, and statements that shame the child should always be avoided by staff members.

Other therapies include individual psychotherapy designed to help the child more appropriately manage the conflict and anger resulting from inadequately resolved separation-individuation issues. Family work is critical. Both parent training and family therapy are usually required for successful treatment.

Although medical-behavioral treatment is effective in 80% of cases (Garfinkel 1990; Levine and Bakow 1976), most of our patients who have responded favorably with a significant diminution of symptoms during hospitalization have subsequently presented with at least one episode of encopresis following discharge. Ongoing postdischarge individual and family therapies are necessary to consolidate and build on gains made during hospitalization.

Anorexia Nervosa

Although anorexia nervosa is much more common in adolescents, it does occur in latency-age children. Five of the last 300 children admitted to our university unit have had anorexia nervosa. Yates' (1990) excellent review of the treatment and outcome for these patients clearly outlines inpatient treatment phases.

Patient stabilization and weight gain are the first objectives. An initial diet of 1,200 to 1,500 calories a day is initiated and increased weekly by 500 calories to a total of approximately 3,000 calories per day. Tube feeding should be used only as a last resort. Hyperalimentation should be avoided because of the high rate of associated morbidity (Andersen et al. 1985).

Nutritional counseling with a dietitian helps determine the patient's ideal weight as well as the weight necessary for discharge. A gradual gain of 2–3 pounds per week is the goal. Behavioral modification techniques, especially social activity reinforcers, are used to augment food intake. Attendance at social activities depends on patient compliance. Bathroom usage is monitored for 2 hours following meals to discourage vomiting.

Once stabilized, other therapies are considered. Family therapy is often essential for generalization of hospital gains following discharge. Although family dysfunction ought not be assumed in all cases (Vandereycken 1987; Yates 1990), many prepubertal anorexic girls develop symptoms in response to family and environmental pressures. These issues must be understood and explored and often require either a structural approach or an object-relations family therapy approach. The latter is more suitable if narcissistic or borderline character structures are evident in family members. Individual psychotherapy used to initially establish an alliance (Andersen et al. 1985) should eventually help the patient identify and understand the internal conflicts and struggle for autonomy that are acted out through the symptoms (Bruch 1973; Yates 1990).

Pharmacotherapy is useful when anorexia coexists with other diagnostic entities that have been shown to respond to medication. Although follow-up data are limited, the tricyclic antidepressants have shown some promise in helping ameliorate depressive symptoms in anorexic girls. Antipsychotic medication should be used with care, and only when other symptoms warrant it (see Chapter 8).

Anorexic patients are often very disruptive within the milieu. Their food refusals, dysthymia, and oppositionalism contribute to inappropriate behaviors by other patients who may either reject them or mistakenly try to nurture them. Their need for monitoring after meals deflects the attention of staff from other patients who then feel resentful. Children who have been raised in very deprived circumstances may be astonished at another child's refusal of food.

Furthermore, these patients create countertransference problems for therapists and child care workers. Chronic anorexic patients are especially difficult because of their intransigence and self-destructive behavior. Therapists sometimes employ more invasive interventions than necessary (e.g., using tube feeding before other reinforcers have been adequately tried) as a response to their own frustration. Supervision and ongoing staff discussion are necessary to guard against staff acting out.

In our experience, it takes 2 to 4 months to adequately treat prepubertal anorexic girls during the hospitalization phase. Although the adolescent literature suggests that half of the successfully treated hospital patients relapse following discharge (Hsu 1980), we have found that the treatment of school-age children is more successful, although there are no studies to support this view. If the hospital treatment team is not going to continue the postdischarge therapy, there must be efficient communication with the posthospitalization therapist to review patient and family symptoms and dynamics, inpatient treatment approaches, and patient response.

Developmental Issues

Preschool Children

The admission of preschool children presents special problems within the milieu. Although preschool children are frequently hospitalized on school-age units, few inpatient studies have investigated this group. In a descriptive report, Buffet-Arinal and Mazet (1982) discussed the use of inpatient transference manifestations to understand family interactional problems. In a recent study, we examined the developmental, family, and community factors that contribute to the hospitalization of preschool children, presenting information about patient symptoms, diagnosis, family situation, and demographic considerations in 18 preschool inpatients (Dalton et al. 1987). The data indicated that most of the preschoolers were hospitalized because their severe symptoms could be neither contained nor successfully treated within their disturbed and unsupportive family settings, and they were not able to be managed in less restrictive out-of-home settings. Furthermore, serious maternal psychopathology and family chaos were associated with psychopathology in the study group.

What differentiates preschool children from school-age children is the comparative immaturity of the younger children. They need ongoing parental support and nurturance even more consistently and predictably than do school-age children. Thus, 3- and 4-year-olds should only be removed from the home if their safety is jeopardized and should only be hospitalized if problematic behaviors cannot be contained in less restrictive settings.

Special consideration must be given to preschool children on the unit. Primary caregivers must be assigned who work diligently to gain trust and to establish an alliance. Nurturance must be provided, especially at times traditionally difficult for young children (e.g., bedtime, unit transitions, times of separation). In fact, our experience is that the remission of symptoms is predicated on both the establishment of an alliance and the provision of nurturance.

Generalization of gains made during the hospital process is very difficult with this group. Our own follow-up data clearly underscore the problems these children encounter following discharge (Dalton et al. 1990). We believe that the hospital process itself potentially contributes to poor long-term outcome. The individual, family, and milieu therapies necessary both to diminish symptoms and to meet developmental needs, combined with the paucity of appropriate community resources, often necessitate extended lengths of stay for these children. The severing of trusting hospital relationships at discharge, even when handled well, creates enormous problems for preschool patients, contributing to internal insecurity and personal wariness about future relationships. We suspect that children who can be successfully treated in short periods of time possess the sort of individual, family, and/or community resources that make hospitalization unnecessary, in spite of recent reports (Mansheim 1990).

Many preschool inpatients are discharged to out-of-home settings because of ongoing family chaos. Sometimes there are multiple posthospital placements, further compromising the development of ongoing attachments.

The optimal out-of-home treatment setting, in lieu of hospitalization, is a small therapeutic group home where patients do not have to be immediately discharged when symptoms remit, allowing for ongoing relationship building as well as for an orderly transition, when possible, back to home. Such settings are expensive, however, and the present economic climate makes their development unlikely. Because psychiatric admissions of very disturbed preschool children to hospitals will probably continue, we suggest that the following four elements are necessary for a successful hospitalization and discharge (Dalton et al. 1987):

1. A special program specifically designed to meet the child's developmental and psychiatric needs is essential.

2. The hospital must be prepared for an extended hospitalization, and plans for discharge must be based on both the resolution of psychiatric symptoms and the state of the child's special unit relationships (i.e., the psychological level of the child's attachments with staff).
3. The posthospital placement must adequately meet the child's special developmental attachment needs and psychiatric needs.
4. The implementation of the discharge plan must take into account the time required for adequate separation from the hospital.

Preteen Children

Some 11- and 12-year-olds requiring hospitalization belong on school-age units, whereas others are more suited for adolescent units. The choice depends on the particular patient's developmental needs. When the needs for dependence and nurturance are the main conflict areas contributing to problematic behavior, school-age units are indicated. When problems involve substance abuse, sexual acting out, peer group conflicts, and behaviors representing independence struggles, an adolescent unit is appropriate. Furthermore, large, physically aggressive preteen children sometimes require an adolescent unit because they physically intimidate smaller children.

Unit workers must closely monitor preteen children for both aggressive and sexual acting out. The intimidation of younger, more vulnerable patients is always a concern. Disturbed preteen children requiring inpatient care who are conflicted about their own dependency needs almost always act out aggressively or sexually, or by disobeying unit rules when other younger patients are receiving appropriate nurturance. This dynamic must be understood and approached therapeutically with the patient. As illustrated in the case example in Chapter 10 of the three preteen children who became aggressive at night, these children tried to hide their needs behind misbehavior, because they felt ashamed of their underlying wishes and fears.

Because of the changing developmental needs of children in this age group (i.e., movement toward independence), child care workers should give these patients appropriate psychological "space" when applying consequences. The rules for school-age children are clearly spelled out, and consequences for infractions of the rules are consistently and predictably applied. With adolescents, the rules are clearly stated, but the application of consequences must take into account developmental issues. Instead of an immediate application of consequences, adolescents are asked to join the process by understanding what they have done and by voluntarily accepting previously negotiated consequences. This approach is necessary to both maintain unit structure and enhance the adolescent's sense of developing autonomy. With preteen children, child care workers strike a balance between the immediate application of consequences and encouraging these children to accept previously discussed limits. For example, when a latency-age child acts out sufficiently to require time out, that limit is immediately set. If the child refuses, child care workers explain that the patient will be held until he or she is able to comply. With preteen children, however, child care workers respond to inappropriate behavior by verbally indicating the previously chosen consequence. If the preteen child scoffs, the child care worker encourages the patient to accept the consequences, but does not immediately enforce them physically. This gives the preteen patient a "face-saving" opportunity that is developmentally appropriate. If the preteen patient continues to refuse after a reasonable period of time, however, the consequences are then enforced.

References

Achenbach T, Edelbrock C: Manual for the Child Behavior Checklist and Revised Child Behavior Profile. Burlington, VT, Thomas M Achenbach, 1983

Alessi NE, Magen J: Panic disorder in psychiatrically hospitalized children. Am J Psychiatry 145:1450–1452, 1988

American Academy of Child and Adolescent Psychiatry: Guidelines for the clinical evaluation of child and adolescent sexual abuse. J Am Acad Child Adolesc Psychiatry 27:655–657, 1988

American Psychiatric Association: Diagnostic and Statistical Manual of Mental Disorders, 3rd Edition, Revised. Washington, DC, American Psychiatric Association, 1987

Andersen AE, Morse CL, Santmyer KS: Inpatient treatment for anorexia nervosa, in Handbook of Psychotherapy for Anorexia Nervosa and Bulimia. Edited by Garner DM, Garfinkel PE. New York, Guilford, 1985, pp 311–343

Brent D, Kolko DJ: Suicide and suicidal behavior in children and adolescents, in Psychiatric Disorders in Children and Adolescents. Edited by Garfinkel B, Carlson G, Weller E. Philadelphia, PA, WB Saunders, 1990, pp 372–391

Bruch H: Eating Disorders: Obesity and Anorexia Nervosa. New York, Basic Books, 1973

Buffet-Arinal Y, Mazet P: Psychopathologie du premier age—l'experience d'hospitalisation dans une Unité de soin psychiatriques pour jeune enfant. Neuropsychiatrie de l'Enfance et de l'Adolescence 30:219–223, 1982

Campbell N: Suicidal children and their families. Poster presentation at the annual meeting of the American Academy of Child and Adolescent Psychiatry, Chicago, IL, October 1990

Cantor S, Kestenbaum C: Psychotherapy with schizophrenic children. Journal of the American Academy of Child Psychiatry 25:623–630, 1986

Carlson GA, Asarnow JR, Orbach I: Developmental aspects of suicidal behavior in children, I. J Am Acad Child Adolesc Psychiatry 26:186–192, 1987

Cohen-Sandler R, Berman AL, King RA: A follow-up study of hospitalized suicidal children. Journal of the American Academy of Child Psychiatry 21:398–403, 1982

Dalton R, Haslett N, Daul G: Alternative therapy with a recalcitrant fire-setter. Journal of the American Academy of Child Psychiatry 25:713–717, 1986

Dalton R, Forman M, Daul G, et al: Psychiatric hospitalization of preschool children: admission factors and discharge implications. J Am Acad Child Adolesc Psychiatry 26:308–312, 1987

Dalton R, Bolding D, Forman M: Psychiatric hospitalization of preschool children: a follow-up study. Child Psychiatry Hum Dev 21:57–64, 1990

Deblinger E, McLeer S, Henry D: Cognitive behavioral treatment for sexually abused children suffering post-traumatic stress: preliminary findings. J Am Acad Child Adolesc Psychiatry 29:747–752, 1990

Erikson E: Childhood and Society. New York, WW Norton, 1963

Farber JM: Psychopharmacology of self-injurious behavior in the mentally retarded. J Am Acad Child Adolesc Psychiatry 26:296–302, 1987

Fineman KR: Firesetting in childhood and adolescence. Psychiatr Clin North Am 3:483–500, 1980

Garfinkel B: The elimination disorders, in Psychiatric Disorders in Children and Adolescents. Edited by Garfinkel B, Carlson G, Weller E. Philadelphia, WB Saunders, 1990, pp 325–336

Garrison W: Predicting violent behavior in psychiatrically hospitalized boys. Journal of Youth and Adolescence 13:225–238, 1984

Garrison WT, Ecker B, Friedman M, et al: Aggression and counteraggression during child psychiatric hospitalization. J Am Acad Child Adolesc Psychiatry 29:242–250, 1990

Hsu LKG: Outcome of anorexia nervosa: a review of the literature (1954–1978). Arch Gen Psychiatry 37:1041–1046, 1980

Kohan MJ, Pothier P, Norbeck JS: Hospitalized children with history of sexual abuse: incidence and care issues. Am J Orthopsychiatry 57:258–264, 1987

Kolko DJ, Kazdin AE: Motives of childhood firesetters: firesetting characteristics and psychological correlates. J Child Psychol Psychiatry 32:535–550, 1991

Kovacs M: Rating scales to assess depression in school-aged children. Acta Paediatr Scand 46:306–315, 1980

Levine M, Bakow H: Children with encopresis: a study of treatment outcome. Pediatrics 58:845–852, 1976

Lewis DO, Lewis M, Unger L, et al: Conduct disorder and its synonyms: diagnoses of dubious validity and usefulness. Am J Psychiatry 141:514–519, 1984

Mansheim P: Short-term psychiatric inpatient treatment of preschool children. Hosp Community Psychiatry 41:670–672, 1990

McLeer SV, Deblinger E, Atkins MS, et al: Post-traumatic stress disorder in sexually abused children. J Am Acad Child Adolesc Psychiatry 27:650–654, 1988

Myers WC, Carrera F III: Carbamazepine-induced mania with hypersexuality in a 9-year-old boy. Am J Psychiatry 146:400, 1989

Pfeffer CR: The Suicidal Child. New York, Guilford, 1986

Pfeffer CR, Plutchik R, Mizruchi MS: Suicidal and assaultive behaviors in children: classification, measurements, and interrelations. Am J Psychiatry 140:154–157, 1983

Pfeffer CR, Plutchik R, Mizruchi MS, et al: Assaultive behavior in child psychiatric inpatients, outpatients, and nonpatients. J Am Acad Child Adolesc Psychiatry 26:256–261, 1987

Spielberger C: Preliminary Manual for the State-Trait Anxiety Inventory for Children. Palo Alto, CA, Consulting Psychologists, 1973

Stewart MA, Culver KW: Children who set fires: the clinical picture and a follow-up. Br J Psychiatry 140:357–363, 1982

Vandereycken W: The constructive family approach to eating disorders: critical remarks on the use of family therapy in anorexia nervosa and bulimia. International Journal of Eating Disorders 6:455–467, 1987

Werry JS, Wollersheim JP: Behavior therapy with children and adolescents: a twenty-year overview. J Am Acad Child Adolesc Psychiatry 28:1–18, 1989

Wysocki R: Behavioral pharmacology and self-injury, in Advances in the Treatment of Self-Injurious Behavior. Edited by Griffin J, Stark M, Williams D, et al. Austin, TX, Texas Planning Council for Developmental Disabilities, 1984

Yates A: Current perspectives on the eating disorders, II: treatment, outcome, and research directions. J Am Acad Child Adolesc Psychiatry 29:1–9, 1990

Chapter 14

School

Although considered a necessary component of overall inpatient treatment, school-age unit school programs are very sparsely represented in the literature. As Blotcky and Lichtenstein (1986) indicate, inpatient school programs have emphasized the need for coordination and interrelatedness between school and milieu personnel. In this chapter we review the various administrative school designs for inpatient care, two classroom models frequently used, the importance of effective coordination of the school program with the treatment program, and the role of the teacher.

There are five basic goals for inpatient participation in an ongoing school process (Table 14–1). The first is to help patients develop ego strengths (Stone 1979). School provides an opportunity for children to work toward stated goals with the help of a teacher and child care worker. Accomplishments, especially during times of emotional flux, help build confidence, a sense of self-efficacy, and self-esteem. Second, classroom experience provides an opportunity for the assessment of each patient's academic level, academic potential, and school behavior. Typically, the classroom is a place where conflicted latency-age children act out. Both the group experience and the emphasis on performance can negatively affect some children, leading to various disruptive and inappropriate behaviors like those precipitating hospitalization. The data derived from the inpatient classroom setting contribute valuable information to the overall evaluation process and subsequent treatment planning. Third, the unit school program offers an opportunity for continued learning by patients during hospitalization. A fourth goal is the evaluation and the provision of services for children with special academic and educational needs. Finally, inpatient educational programs assist in the generalization of inpatient gains to post-discharge settings.

Coordination between the school and the milieu is critical for the attainment of these goals. Interrelatedness and efficient communication be-

Table 14–1. Five basic goals for inpatient participation in an ongoing unit school process

To help patients develop ego strengths
To provide an opportunity for the assessment of each patient's academic level, academic potential, and school behavior
To offer an opportunity for continued learning by patients during the hospitalization process
To identify and evaluate children with special academic and educational needs and provide services
To assist in the generalization of inpatient gains to the various postdischarge settings

tween the teacher and other team members are necessary to ensure that the same behavioral techniques used within the milieu are also used in the classroom. Furthermore, a close working relationship between teacher and milieu staff imparts a sense of security to the patients and discourages psychological splitting.

Several potential problems confound communication and coordination between school and unit staff. There are basic differences in the manner in which childhood anxiety and psychopathology are managed by school and psychiatric personnel (Hirschberg 1953). Traditionally, teachers seldom offer interpretations. They support defenses instead of offering insight to their use, and they deal in the here and now instead of taking both a situational and a historical perspective. In short, teachers have different (at times competing) short-term goals in their work with children than do inpatient clinicians. It is important that mental health staff be aware that this traditional stance of teachers need not be a threat to their own work with patients and is similar to what the child will encounter in the postdischarge school setting. However, when school personnel refuse to join the overall treatment process, care becomes disjointed, leading to acrimony between school and unit personnel.

On the other hand, the role of the inpatient teacher can become blurred. Teachers sometimes see themselves as psychotherapists, consequently altering their more traditional approaches and thus confusing the patients.

Staffings, team meetings, and informal discussions provide the means for the necessary coordination. The unit medical director and team leader must each make a special effort to work with the teacher and school personnel. They should clearly spell out patient and family dynamics in a way that clarifies the purposes of specific milieu interventions. Their work is directed toward developing a consensus on which behavioral interventions should be used during classroom work.

Size

The size of the unit school, including the number of students and the number of classes, has an important bearing on how the education program functions. Single classroom inpatient programs are used when there is a minimal number of patients and are typically found on small units in university and general hospitals. This particular design enhances coordination and communication. However, it calls for a teacher who is comfortable working concurrently with students at various academic levels.

Multiple classrooms are necessary to meet the needs of large inpatient programs in psychiatric hospitals with several adolescent and school-age units. A principal is usually necessary to organize and manage the teaching effort. Of course, increased coordination and communication are required because of the number of students, teachers, and unit personnel involved. If well developed, however, a large program can provide a more sophisticated, varied educational design not possible with fewer personnel.

Administration

There are two possible sources of administrative control over the school program. The local or state school system often provides teachers and administrative personnel for state psychiatric hospitals and, in some school districts, for all other hospitals with school-age or adolescent psychiatric units. The choice of curriculum, hiring of teachers, and formation of general school policy are handled by the public school district administration. Discharge educational planning is facilitated by the use of this administrative model, especially when the child is returning to a home-based school located within the same district as the hospital school. However, the unit medical director or hospital administrator has no authority to select or supervise the teachers, or to remove a teacher if performance is unsatisfactory and treatment is undermined. Furthermore, increased coordination is required to manage splitting by patients or families—a frequent consequence of this model.

Many for-profit hospitals, children's hospitals, and university hospitals with children's units hire their own teachers and school personnel. The administrative control rests within the hospital. This approach significantly enhances the coordination between the unit and classroom, although postdischarge planning is more complicated. There are two basic subtypes, depending on the number of units within a particular hospital. When there is only one unit in the hospital with patients requiring an educational program, administrative control usually rests within the unit with either the unit director or head nurse, depending on the overall administrative structure (see Chapter 15). In hospitals with multiple psychiatric units, administrative control of the school usually rests with the hospital administrator. As reviewed in the next, and final, chapter, this administrative model requires close communication between the unit director and the hospital administrator for smooth functioning.

The Classroom

The classroom model proposed by Blotcky and Lichtenstein (1986) is one of the few presented in the literature. Their program, designed to meet the needs of 12 children, employs one special education teacher and two child care workers.

Each child is placed in school on the day following admission, whenever possible. Evaluation tests, such as the Peabody Individual Achievement Test (PIAT) (Dunn and Markwardt 1970), are used to determine current academic functioning in mathematics, reading, and general information. Based on that information, as well as psychological testing data, an individualized educational plan is devised by the teacher. Weekly lesson plans are subsequently formulated, and necessary classroom materials are gathered. Special emphasis is placed on developing vocabulary, bolstering deficit areas, recognizing main ideas, and identifying cause-and-effect relationships. Physical education, music, and occupational therapy are offered. Child care workers assist the special education teacher in supervising both academic achievement and behavior. In this way, highly individualized help is offered amidst a highly structured environment.

Treatment interventions include time out and the removal of children to a quiet room, when necessary. A systemic reinforcement program is used to enhance movement toward academic goals. Homework and daily study hall are also used. Report cards are issued on a 6-week basis. Follow-up data have shown that patients within this system have advanced at an academically favorable rate.

There are other alternatives to the classroom model described above. One or two patients at a time may attend class for several hours per day followed by a structured homework experience with one-to-one staff supervision on the unit. This abbreviated but intensive model focuses on reading and mathematics, after an initial thorough educational evaluation. Some units provide an exclusive home-bound educational experience on the unit itself. Although there is no current research comparing these approaches, it is our experience that the more structured, formal programs provide the most predictable results.

In most models, child care workers accompany patients to the school, where they also function as teacher's aides. This is especially important for behaviorally difficult children. It is necessary to ensure that behavioral interventions used within the milieu are also used within the classroom, that they are applied uniformly, and that children are not routinely returned to the unit when they misbehave. Although there are no studies depicting the ideal teacher-patient ratio for inpatient education programs, it has been our experience that at least one education worker per four patients is necessary for the attainment of modest goals (e.g., one teacher and one child care worker for a class of eight children). A more favorable ratio, however, is often necessary to achieve complex goals and objectives. Of course, appropriate educational equipment and materials are especially necessary for optimal results.

The Teacher

Teachers basically need the same strengths and talents required of other unit workers. In addition, they must be flexible enough to work within a system different from their own. They must be able to balance educational goals with treatment goals, helping the team understand how symptoms both impact on and are a product of school functioning.

Assessing learning problems and implementing meaningful, individualized, success-oriented curricula (Blotcky and Lichtenstein 1986) are responsibilities that are also expected of the teachers. In addition, teachers must coordinate their work with unit personnel and supervise unit staff in their educational work with inpatients, such as when patients require tutoring or are assigned homework.

Poorly managed countertransference issues potentially interfere with the work of the teacher. By and large, teachers are not trained to identify how their own basic beliefs, past experiences, and personal defenses influence their responses to patient behavior. Furthermore, they often do not know how to use their own countertransference to better understand patient motivations and transferences. Although the lack of insight regarding countertransference is usually not a problem in traditional school settings, it can become a major issue within a working environment where everyone else is expected to examine their own motives and feelings and to react accordingly.

As previously noted, difficulties occur when the teacher tries to also be a therapist. Teaching is different from psychotherapy. When teachers begin to use interpretation and other therapeutic techniques, they expectedly engender patient anxiety that distracts the child from the work necessary to achieve educational goals and objectives.

Follow-up

Coordination between the unit school and the postdischarge educational placement occupies a major part of the discharge plan. Both the teacher and the clinician should contact the future school to discuss the patient's academic achievement and behavior in the classroom. The child's specific academic level in each educational skill (e.g., mathematics, reading) is clearly stated so that immediate placement at the correct level is possible following discharge. Furthermore, successful behavioral and milieu interventions used during the inpatient stay are discussed in detail. Although the teacher should have the necessary data to reasonably inform the home-based school about these matters, it is the clinician who must take the responsibility to make sure that appropriate liaison work occurs. Alexson and Sinclair (1986) have shown that inpatients tend to receive a higher percentage of changes to more restrictive educational settings following discharge than do outpatients who carry the same diagnoses following evaluation. Overly restrictive postdischarge placements can be just as deleterious to long-term outcome as are inadequately structured placements. The clinician should work with the home-based teachers, counselors, and principal to make sure that they do not overestimate the patient's psychopathology and offer an unnecessarily restrictive program, thereby reinforcing the child's already lowered sense of self-esteem. For many children their inpatient school experience has represented their first educational success.

References

Alexson J, Sinclair E: Psychiatric diagnosis and school placement: a comparison between inpatients and outpatients. Child Psychiatry Hum Dev 16:194–205, 1986

Blotcky M, Lichtenstein A: Integration of education in child residential treatment. Residential Treatment for Children and Youth 4:41–49, 1986

Dunn L, Markwardt F: Peabody Individual Achievement Test. Circle Pines, MN, American Guidance Service, 1970

Hirschberg JC: The education of emotionally disturbed children, 4: the role of education in the treatment of emotionally disturbed children through planned ego development. Am J Orthopsychiatry 23:684–690, 1953

Stone L: Residential treatment, in Basic Handbook of Child Psychiatry, Vol 3: Therapeutic Interventions. Edited by Harrison SI (JD Noshpitz, Editor-in-Chief). New York, Basic Books, 1979, pp 231–262

Chapter 15

Administration and Interfaces

Administrative Models

Models of administration describe the specific hospital unit organizational plans used for carrying out and executing the goals of hospitalization. Administrative models operate both at the level of the clinical treatment team and at the level of the unit as a whole. Two discrete but related administrative structures underlie all child inpatient services. The *clinical team* consists of all therapists, nurses, and child care workers involved in the collection and evaluation of diagnostic data and the provision of therapy for a particular child. The *unit administration* consists of the individuals involved in the direction, organization, and maintenance of both the unit and the milieu. On well-functioning units, the algorithms supporting each are understood, accepted, and well coordinated.

Clinical Team Administration

Noshpitz (1975) has outlined three types of administration of clinical teams. The *team-oriented (TO) approach* emphasizes communication among all team members (Rinsley 1980). Each team member performs predetermined evaluation and treatment tasks and is administratively and clinically responsible to a supervisor who is not part of the specific clinical team. The team leader (usually, but not always, a psychiatrist) chairs meetings. He or she is responsible for organizing the treatment plan and suggests specific evaluation and treatment approaches, but does not have the administrative authority to ensure compliance. The team leader's authority is primarily sapiential, based on training and knowledge (Geraty 1989). Efficient clinical functioning often depends on the leader's ability to effectively convey reasonable ideas, the alliance among the leader and team members, and the team members' abilities to implement their parts of the treatment plan.

The *authority-oriented (AO) approach* emphasizes the leader's power and authority. The leader chairs meetings and staffings. He or she is responsible for the organization of the treatment plan, assigns clinicians to perform certain evaluation and treatment tasks, and supervises clinical work. Each team member answers directly to the leader, who is responsible for orchestrating the entire process.

The *therapist-centered (TC) team approach,* originally used in traditional psychiatric hospitals during the 1940s and 1950s, emphasizes the importance of the individual psychotherapist. This administrative design is poorly centralized, and communication among team members is deemphasized. Goals and objectives for hospitalization and discharge criteria are determined by the therapist, while daily living issues are managed by nurses or milieu coordinators. The importance of patient functioning within the milieu is minimized, in contrast to the patient's progress in therapy.

In addition to these different types of team administrations, clinical services vary according to the number of treatment teams working within specific units. Some units have only one functioning clinical treatment team, while others have multiple teams. Furthermore, these multiple teams are sometimes chaired by leaders who work closely together (i.e., group practice partners), while, in other situations, the teams are unrelated.

Unit Administration

Although there are a number of ways of conceptualizing various children's unit administrative styles, in our opinion these styles are most clearly illustrated by understanding the role of the medical director (i.e., the unit director) within each example.

Licensing and accreditation agencies require that each children's unit have a medical director charged with the responsibilities of ensuring that all patients satisfy stated admission criteria and of supervising general clinical and medical services. Nevertheless, the power and authority of the medical director differs significantly in different administrative models, which in turn are based on hospital policy and administrative philosophy. However, the courts have made it clear that the medical director will be held responsible for the medical and clinical services offered within the unit regardless of the power and authority granted the director within any given hospital. Thus, the medical director must be comfortable with the specific administrative structure and treatment philosophy of the employing institution (Geraty 1989).

Regardless of the administrative model, the medical director needs to have well-developed clinical, managerial, and interpersonal skills. Planning, organizing, staffing, directing, communicating, and providing control and innovation are vital skills (Harper and Geraty 1987). Knowing when to be assertive and when to be conciliatory is also important. These skills are rarely acquired in training, but are usually a product of experience and temperament. In our opinion, the medical director should be a child psychiatrist who works at least half-time in this capacity for units of 8 to 10 beds, and full-time for units of 15 to 20 beds.

Matrix model. The matrix model approach to unit administration describes shared authority and power. There are two basic examples, the first describing shared authority between two people, usually the medical director and the head nurse. In the *dual matrix model* (DM), the medical director oversees all clinical services necessary to accomplish the goals of hospitalization. The head nurse is responsible for the actual milieu structure and staff members' behavior within the unit (e.g., establishing rules for unit workers, supervising worker behavior, disciplinary action). The head nurse also monitors the hospital accreditation guidelines and standards as they pertain to the unit. Coordination between these two individuals is vital for successful unit functioning. Optimal clinical performance is unlikely unless the medical director and head nurse clearly understand and accept their roles, communicate effectively, and actively support each other. Both are responsible to the hospital administrator, who ideally is well informed about unit functioning although usually not directly involved.

The second unit matrix design, the *multiple matrix model* (MM), consists of multiple lines of shared authority. The head nurse is responsible for the nurses on the unit, the milieu coordinator for the child care workers and implementation of the milieu plan, the medical director for psychiatric services, and the unit chief psychologist and social worker for their respective clinical services. Each may answer to a different individual within the hospital administration—for example, the unit head nurse reports to the director of nursing, the unit social worker to the director of social work, and so forth.

There are two variations of this multiple matrix model, one with a relatively strong medical director and the other without. A "strong" medical director has the authority, delegated by the hospital administrator, to monitor each component of clinical care within the unit (milieu, nursing service, individual treatment teams, activities therapy, etc.) and to make suggestions for appropriate changes that will, in most cases, be implemented. A "weak" medical director has no such administrative support and thus can only comment on various components of clinical care, but has very little clout and is thus usually unable to affect reasonable change.

Hierarchical model. The hierarchical model (H) is different from the matrix approach in that there is a single line of authority, the medical director, on the unit. That individual is responsible for overseeing all clinical services as well as for the actual governance of the unit, the milieu, and the staff. The medical director within this model answers directly to the hospital administrator. The model is rather antiquated, dating back to a previous era when the other disciplines had less well-defined professional identities and were more subservient to the orders of the physician.

Combining Team and Unit Administrations

The three clinical team models are combined with specific unit administrative models. The dual matrix model works best with the authority-oriented clinical team approach (DM-AO) especially when there is only one clinical team that serves all the children on the unit. In this combination, the unit medical director is also chairperson of the clinical treatment team. The main advantage that accrues from this model is that admissions, evaluations, therapies, research, and training can be effectively coordinated and monitored. It fosters a focused treatment plan approach, so that each patient's needs will be addressed. The main potential disadvantage is a product of the reduced number of checks and balances implicit on a unit combining the medical director and clinical team leader roles. This situation is successfully avoided on units where the child psychiatrist, head nurse, psychologist, and social worker develop a trusting relationship that encourages open discussion of treatment planning. This model is used primarily on small units within university and children's hospitals.

The multiple matrix administrative unit model with a relatively strong medical director is often combined with the team-oriented clinical team approach (MM-TO). This combination is frequently seen on large state hospital units with many patients but with few resources. The unit medical director serves also as chairman of the treatment team, oftentimes for as many as 20 to 25 patients. Although each member of the team is officially supervised by clinicians and administrators not directly involved in day-to-day unit functioning, the medical director also supervises clinical services and generally has the authority to modify particular evaluation and treatment approaches according to perceived patient need.

The chief advantages and disadvantages of this combination are related. Because the medical director, who is also the team leader in this model, has multiple responsibilities and many patients, he or she is usually too busy to personally direct each component of each patient's evaluation and therapy. This disadvantage is lessened by the team members' predetermined responsibilities for particular segments of the diagnostic and treatment process. Frequently, a case manager chosen from among team members is appointed to monitor each patient's response to the provision of clinical services and movement toward satisfying the discharge criteria. Although this sometimes creates an assembly line–like approach, it does reasonably ensure that patient needs will not be overlooked.

The relationship between the hospital administration and the medical director, important in all models, is especially vital here. If team members and administrative and clinical supervisors understand that the medical director–team leader has the support of the hospital administrator, the chances for psychological splitting and undermining of the medical director's authority are reduced. The medical director must establish an alliance with each team member and off-unit supervisor so that both clinical and staff matters can be managed without untoward unit discord.

The multiple matrix administrative model in which the medical director has very little authority is frequently combined with the authority-oriented clinical team approach (MM-AO) on school-age units with multiple teams (usually within private and for-profit hospitals). Here, the medical director is a titular head, necessary to satisfy accreditation needs, or sometimes used to troubleshoot by the hospital administrator, but without much authority to affect substantive change within the unit. The multiple clinical teams are chaired by private practice psychiatrists who have any number of patients on the unit at one time. Members of the team answer directly to the team leader.

An advantage of this model is that it can introduce to one unit several highly trained, competent clinicians. Patients can be diagnosed and treated very efficiently, especially if the treatment team is not responsible for large numbers of patients. The major disadvantage of this combination often affects the milieu, however. The type of coordination necessary for effective unitwide programs that include parent management training, behavioral management within the milieu, group therapy, and research is very difficult with multiple teams. Private practitioners frequently do not have the time to meet and discuss issues not directly related to their own patients. Unless the hospital provides a milieu coordinator responsible for maintaining communication with each team leader, patient and parental acting out and splitting are likely to occur.

On well-functioning units employing this model, a number of these potential problems are handled in medical staff meetings where clinicians have the opportunity to both confront hospital administrators with possible unit shortcomings and organize themselves in order to better coordinate unit care for their patients. This task is easier to accomplish when the clinicians know and respect each other and have experience working together.

The hierarchical administrative unit model was used in combination with the therapist-centered treatment approach (H-TC) in traditional psychiatric hospital units when individual therapy was the primary, and often exclusive, treatment and when patient cure was the goal.

The hierarchical model is currently used in tandem with the authority-oriented treatment team (H-AO) in some state hospital and private units. This approach places extraordinary responsibility on the medical director with few checks and balances. It can work quite effectively with a competent, motivated medical director, but can be a disaster in the wrong hands.

The various combinations of team and unit administration are summarized in Figure 15–1.

Relationship Between the Medical Director and the Hospital Administrator

The collaborative relationship between the unit medical director and the hospital administrator can affect the functioning of the unit. If they respect one another and work together well, difficult problems can be handled in a satisfactory manner. In our experience, there are four troublesome issues that can disrupt this relationship and adversely affect the unit:

1. Conflicts regarding admission policies and procedures
2. Disagreements about staffing patterns and unit supplies
4. Matrix system problems
4. Concerns about families whose ability to pay for inpatient care is disrupted before the need for hospitalization is over

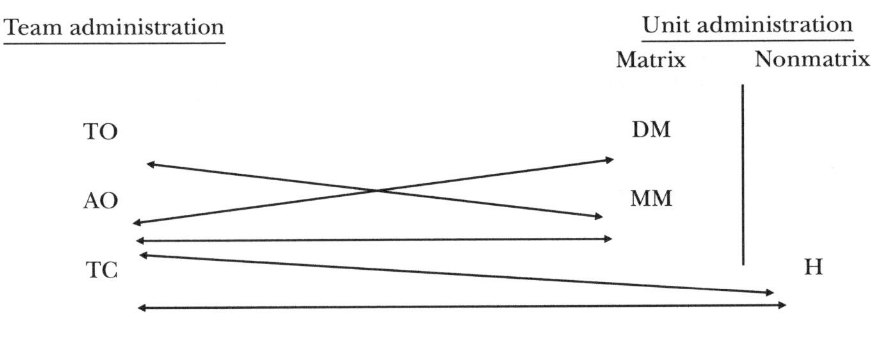

Figure 15–1. Combinations of team-unit administration. TO = team-oriented approach; AO = authority-oriented approach; TC = therapist-centered team approach; DM = dual matrix model; MM = multiple matrix model; H = heirarchical model.

Some admission practices, as discussed in Chapter 2, present problems for clinicians and unit staff in both private and public hospitals. These include 1) the inappropriate admission by market-driven emergency assessment teams of patients who might be successfully treated in less restrictive settings; 2) uncoordinated admissions to public units by mental health professionals who work outside the hospital; and 3) an increased number of new admissions to a unit within a short period of time.

It is the medical director's responsibility to monitor how admissions affect milieu functioning. For example, a unit with many aggressive children might not be able to reasonably absorb an additional patient with aggressive symptoms. At the time the patient presents for admission, the medical director should ideally contact both the admitting clinician and the hospital administrator, advising that alternate arrangements should be considered (i.e., a delay of the admission or, if necessary, admission of the child to a unit in another hospital). These situations are most difficult when they negatively affect hospital and clinician income and when other reasonable clinical options are not available. A strong alliance among the decision-makers is essential for the most appropriate clinical decision to be made.

Staffing patterns and the provision of unit supplies are another area of concern that must often be negotiated between the unit director and hospital administration. Because one of the major hospital expenses is staff salaries, administrators are often tempted to cut costs by treating as many patients with as few child care workers and nursing staff members as possible. This unstated policy can lead to obvious difficulties when there are aggressive, acting-out, or suicidal patients who require one-to-one staffing on the unit. More subtle problems result from inadequate staff time to provide necessary nurturance and activities, both of which are vital components of milieu therapy. The medical director must advocate for unit and patient needs with the hospital administrator, clearly and firmly detailing how many milieu staff members are necessary to implement specific components of individual treatment plans and the milieu plan in general.

Multiple matrix system problems may occur, because psychological splitting by patients and staff is always a possibility when multiple individuals are responsible for different services. The hospital administrator, or the administrator's delegate, may need to mediate disagreements within the unit. It is crucial that a smooth working relationship exist between the medical director and hospital administrator so that fair, informed decisions can be made and any subsequent negative feelings discussed.

A fourth compelling reason for a productive working alliance among the medical director, hospital administrators, and individual clinicians involves the financial needs of individual patients. A major obstacle to contemporary psychiatric inpatient practice is the patient's inability to pay for services. Frequently, the patient's source of funding runs out before the inpatient treatment goals are achieved. As discussed in Chapter 6, we believe that it is the responsibility of the clinicians and the hospital to continue the inpatient treatment until objectives have been sufficiently satisfied so that continued developmental and therapeutic gains are possible in a less restrictive setting. The kind of negotiations necessary to implement this policy is predicated on a productive, trusting working alliance among the parties involved.

Confounding Issues

Clinical directors of inpatient units have usually not received any prior training in administration. They may assume administrative responsibilities immediately upon graduation from residency training, or they may be more seasoned clinicians who have "grown into" unit director positions by virtue of experience. In their prior training, which is likely to have been heavily biased toward individual pathology and treatment, courses in group dynamics, organizational theory, and management may be lacking. Residency program directors are now becoming more aware of the need for formal training in administration for residents, but most graduates are truly novices in this area.

The unit director may be viewed by the staff as an omniscient parent, with the unrealistic expectation that he or she can readily solve problems related not only to the patients, but to staffing and budget. The director in turn may feel vulnerable and view the staff as dependent, ungrateful children. Such misperceptions may not be overtly recognized or acknowledged, but rather may be disguised in conflicts between unit director and staff regarding the management of individual patients.

The unit director may at times feel isolated and burdened with a sense of potentially overwhelming responsibility for so many disturbed children on the unit. The director must forge working alliances with staff rather then view himself or herself as the solitary leader; consultation with other inpatient directors may provide useful support and instruction. Despite the frustration inherent in the role, the unit director may also find that the work is quite gratifying. To create and maintain a therapeutic environment for troubled children is not easy, but when accomplished, everyone—director, staff, and patients—will have the sense of a job well done.

Interfaces

As part of the unit and team administrative responsibilities, the medical director and individual clinicians are often required to relate to other physicians, especially pediatricians, to the community, to third-party payers, to the welfare department, to hospital quality assurance, and to trainees in various disciplines. The same alliance-building and interpersonal skills necessary for work with patients are important in these interfaces.

Interface With Pediatrics

As discussed in Chapter 5, pediatricians are frequently consulted to assist in clinical diagnosis and management of medical illnesses. In these cases, the relationship between the child psychiatrist and the pediatrician is usually well defined, with little room for ambiguity. Potential problems may arise, however, when both disciplines are treating inpatients with complex psychological and physical illnesses, as illustrated by the following case of an 11-year-old girl with cystic fibrosis and anorexia nervosa:

> Jane, who had been followed and treated by her pediatrician since infancy for cystic fibrosis, was admitted to our university unit with a diagnosis of anorexia nervosa following a precipitous loss of one-fourth of her weight over a period of 6 weeks. In spite of several hospitalizations for cystic fibrosis, Jane's parents insisted that her condition was mild and that it would not negatively affect her longevity.
>
> Our initial assessment revealed that Jane was unconsciously angry with her parents for denying the reality of her cystic fibrosis. The anorexic symptoms, though multidetermined, served as her attempt to force her family to face the possibility of her own mortality.
>
> It was clear to the treatment team, after talking with Jane's parents and their pediatrician, that neither had broached the question of mortality. The pediatrician had waited for the parents to raise the issue; the parents had assumed that the physician's optimism and reticence about the seriousness of their daughter's illness were good signs. The parents had dealt with their unspoken anxiety about Jane's illness by actively stressing that Jane would have a wonderful future.
>
> The inpatient clinician met with the pediatrician to enlist his assistance in the implementation of the treatment plan. The overall treatment strategy was discussed. The clinician explained how the parents' anxiety over, but denial of, the seriousness of Jane's illness contributed to her psychiatric symptoms. When the pediatrician understood that the parents had to relinquish their fantasy about what Jane was going to be as an adult before their daughter could stop rebelling and refusing to eat, he was able to meet with the parents to realistically discuss the severity of Jane's pulmonary disease. This was an important first step in her overall treatment plan.

This case exemplifies how inpatient clinicians must work with pediatricians and primary care physicians when the patients they work with suffer from illnesses that require concurrent intensive psychiatric and medical management. In order to fully enlist the physician's support, the patient and family dynamics must be explained in a way that makes sense. The primary care physician can then become involved in specific intervention strategies, encouraging active participation in the treatment process.

Interface With the Community

Unit clinicians often speak to community audiences on topics of child development, childhood disorders, parenting techniques, and the impact of various stressors such as divorce, abuse, and parental mental illness, among others. These seminars are usually offered for two purposes: 1) to increase public awareness of childhood issues and 2) to advertise and market hospital programs. These seminars are most effective when speakers concentrate on imparting knowledge about childhood. When the ulterior marketing motive is emphasized more than the educational objectives, the program's potential benefits are diminished.

Overly seductive marketing practices enticing parents to hospitalize children by instilling fear or by subtly promising personality changes not possible during hospitalization make subsequent alliance building with parents and patients very difficult. The unit director and clinicians should monitor hospital promotional practices for accuracy and respond to hospital administrators accordingly.

Interface With the Joint Commission on Accreditation of Healthcare Organizations

All psychiatric inpatient care is now monitored by the Joint Commission on Accreditation of Healthcare Organizations (JCAHO) according to the same standards used for all general hospital treatment and services. Particular attention is paid to dietetic services, emergency services, infection control, medical records, the medical staff, nursing care, pharmaceutical services, safety management, social services, and quality assurance and utilization review (Joint Commission on Accreditation of Healthcare Organizations 1990).

Following the survey in which JCAHO staff visit the hospital seeking accreditation or reaccreditation, the gathered information is forwarded to the Accreditation Committee of the Board of Commissioners of the JCAHO for a decision. The hospital is then accredited with or without type I recommendations (i.e., recommendations for change that must receive the highest priority by the hospital before the next review), conditionally accredited (i.e., immediate changes are necessary), or not accredited.

Nonaccreditation has a profound effect on hospital functioning that, in most circumstances, leads to discontinuation of hospital services and, ultimately, closure of the facility. Some state facilities, totally supported by state funds, escape closure when accreditation is denied.

The weeks leading up to the survey are often hectic for hospital and unit administrators. Time spent managing last-minute details and anxiety about the forthcoming survey often interfere with patient care. This should be monitored closely to limit deleterious effects on unit functioning.

Interface With Quality Assurance

The JCAHO mandates that each hospital must have a quality assurance (QA) program to identify problems in patient care and to resolve them (James 1990; JCAHO 1990). The required characteristics of the program include 1) the establishment of a governing body to ensure the provision of quality patient care hospitalwide; 2) the use of clinical and administrative staffs to resolve identified problems and to communicate their findings and work to the governing body; 3) the establishment of a written plan encompassing the scope of the QA program; and 4) the coordination of the program with risk management within the hospital. Medical staff functions (e.g., monthly meetings, drug usage evaluation, medical record review) and hospitalwide functions (e.g., infection control, utilization review) are detailed within each QA plan. In addition, a systematic way of identifying and responding to problems must be carefully spelled out.

Hospital QA personnel collaborate with unit staff to identify problem areas that interfere with quality of care and to monitor proposed corrective strategies. On our university unit, environmental (e.g., activities, locations, times of day), staff, and patient variables that are related to unit accidents, suicide attempts, aggression, sexual acting out, and group discord are discerned. Subsequent changes in unit schedule, staffing, and patient care are made through proactive planning. QA reviews also examine timeliness of admission physical examinations, factors related to "AMA" (against medical advice) discharges, and parental informed consent for pharmacotherapy, among other measures of quality care. QA should not be viewed as an intrusion into the work of the unit, but rather as a useful mechanism for staff development, improvement in clinical care, and the identification of research questions.

Interface With Third-Party Payers

With the rapid growth of managed health care, insurance benefits for private psychiatric hospitalization have become carefully regulated and, in many instances, dramatically reduced. Payers have moved to control expenditures by establishing arbitrary admission criteria, by mandating fixed lengths of stay for various disorders, and by implementing ongoing external utilization review processes that certify hospitalization on a week-by-week (and sometimes day-by-day) basis.

Utilization review is the process of planning, organizing, and controlling the provision of health care to make it as cost-effective as possible (Connor et al. 1983). It accomplishes its goals primarily by controlling inpatient admissions, lengths of stay, and the use of ancillary services (Zusman 1990). The actual process was introduced into psychiatry during the mid-1970s when the American Psychiatric Association (APA) agreed to provide utilization review for the Civilian Health and Medical Program of the Uniform Services (CHAMPUS) (Hoge 1990), although the APA's peer review process initiated during the 1960s led the way. Today there is both internal and external utilization review. The JCAHO has mandated that each hospital must undertake its own utilization review ideally to improve quality care. Third-party payers, however, basically use utilization review to control their expenses.

Zusman's (1990) description of the current external utilization review system clearly outlines how it functions. At the first level (i.e., screening), cases are mechanically "screened" to determine whether the presenting behaviors and symptoms represent diagnoses that are suitable for admission. Those cases that do not satisfy predetermined (but often unstated) criteria are reviewed at a second level, usually by nurses with clinical experience who review clinical charts or information obtained during telephone interviews with the clinician. If this process does not lead to certification, a third-level review is undertaken by physicians. In addition to this certification process, there is an ongoing concurrent review of the patient's need for continued hospitalization throughout the process, with emphasis on discharge planning.

Zusman and others (Feldstein et al. 1988) question the effectiveness of this process. Current problems with the system include possible denial of services, retrospective refusal of claims leading to mounting debt by families who thought that they were insured, and possible violations of patient confidentiality. Current benefits include cost containment and limitations on unnecessary hospitalizations. There are, as yet, few studies demonstrating the effectiveness of the entire utilization review process (Zusman 1990). In our opinion, it is too soon to determine whether the benefits outweigh the negative side effects.

Clinicians and parents must be aware of, and discuss the limitations of, the particular third-party coverage prior to the formulation of the hospitalization treatment plan. The clinician should consider whether an effective hospitalization treatment plan can be devised within the imposed limitations. Often, the team is forced to focus the treatment planning process on a single problem that, if appropriately handled, can lead to a substantial change in the patient-environment fit so that postdischarge progress will be possible. In many cases, the allotted inpatient time is insufficient to significantly improve the fit. In those cases the family should be referred to a public facility where adequate care is available, or the clinician and hospital administrator may decide in advance to waive fees and costs when the benefits expire.

Frustration with the policies and procedures of the payers and reviewers and subsequently developed countertransference should not be allowed to contaminate the therapeutic relationship with the family (Gabbard et al. 1991). It is appropriate that the family be encouraged to take a proactive stance with their insurer when quality of care is threatened.

Interface With Office of Community Services/Welfare Department

Clinicians work closely with case workers for patients who are in state custody. As soon as discharge criteria have been established and posthospitalization placement needs elucidated, the clinician meets with the case worker to detail short-term and long-term patient needs. Potential complications include workers who are not thoroughly familiar with assigned cases, the inherent slowness of decision making in a state bureaucracy, and the inability of the public system to provide reasonable posthospitalization settings to meet patient needs. Clinicians continually monitor patient progress and, when necessary, contact case worker supervisors directly to facilitate the efficient movement toward fulfilling treatment objectives.

Clinicians are involved with child protective services when their patients have been recently abused or neglected. Sometimes, abuse and neglect are not discovered until the hospitalization process has ensued. At that time clinicians try to enlist parental cooperation in the process, phoning child protection in the presence of parents, or asking the parents to make the call. The clinician strives to maintain the working alliance with parents while at the same time complying with the law.

Interface With Unit Trainees

Child psychiatry residents, medical students, psychology interns, social work students, nursing students, and various allied health trainees are assigned to school-age units for training. Although the purposes for training depend on the goals within each professional discipline, generally they include the development of competence with the various inpatient evaluation and treatment techniques, an understanding of the nature of the milieu and how to use it beneficially, and an appreciation of how the administrative unit format affects clinical functioning. The main problem related to trainees is that they join the milieu often without knowing how to relate to patients with special needs. Thus, they require close, individual supervision, not only for didactic purposes but also to ensure that they do not overidentify with patients or react inappropriately to patient splitting and acting out. Trainees frequently develop close and important relationships with patients; this must be considered when both trainees and patients terminate from the unit. Because of the intensity of the experience, as contrasted with outpatient work, a training rotation on an inpatient service can have a lasting impact on career choice and development.

References

Connor M, Mack G, Handelman E: Dynamics of Utilization Management. Chicago, IL, American Hospital Publishing, 1983

Feldstein P, Wickizer T, Wheeler J: Private cost containment. N Engl J Med 318:1310–1314, 1988

Gabbard GO, Takahashi T, Davidson J, et al: A psychodynamic perspective on the clinical impact of insurance review. Am J Psychiatry 148:318–323, 1991

Geraty R: Administrative issues in inpatient child and adolescent psychiatry. J Am Acad Child Adolesc Psychiatry 28:21–25, 1989

Harper G, Geraty R: Hospital and residential treatment (ch 64), in Psychiatry, Vol 2. Edited by Michels R, Cooper AM, Guze SB, et al. Philadelphia, PA, JB Lippincott, 1987

Hoge SK: Utilization review: a house divided. Hosp Community Psychiatry 41:367–368, 1990

James WS: Introducing quality assurance to a state hospital medical staff. Psychiatr Clin North Am 13:25–34, 1990

Joint Commission on Accreditation of Healthcare Organizations: Accreditation Manual for Hospitals, Vol I: Standards. Oakbrook Terrace, IL, Joint Commission on Accreditation of Healthcare Organizations, 1990

Noshpitz JD: Residential treatment of emotionally disturbed children, in American Handbook of Psychiatry, 2nd Edition, Vol 5: Treatment. Edited by Freedman DX, Dyrud JE (S Arieti, Editor-in-Chief). New York, Basic Books, 1975, pp 634–651

Rinsley DB: Principles of therapeutic milieu with children, in Treatment of Emotional Disorders in Children and Adolescents. Edited by Sholevar G, Benson R, Blinder B. New York, SP Medical and Scientific, 1980, pp 191–208

Zusman J: Utilization review: theory, practice, and issues. Hosp Community Psychiatry 41:531–536, 1990

Index

Page numbers printed in **boldface** refer to tables or figures.